Vegetarian Meal Cook Book

Quick and Easy Meals for Organic and Healthy Vegetarian Diet with Over 100 Recipes to Prep your Keto Meals for Home, Office and Weekly Plans

By

Adele Tyler

All trademarks and brands within this book are for clarifying purposes only and are the owned by the owners themselves, not affiliated with this document.

Table Of Contents

Introduction

We all know the well-known proverb that the knowledge is power, and I'm sure we've all learned one or two things about the power of a vegetarian diet over the past few years. These fantastic foods have dominated American and European media and inundated marketing. And while it is great that we are becoming aware of foods that are healthy and capable of improving our longevity and healing our bodies, there is one crucial factor that was overlooked during the takeover of superfoods.

I just took this upon myself to learn how to cook with superfood as a nutritionist and a home chef. I didn't want to give up my favorite meals. Still, I wanted to practice what I'm preaching to my customers every day. If you treat your body like the super-powered machine, it's, you'll understand why eating quality foods packed with beneficial vitamins, minerals, nutrients, and antioxidants regularly is so important; in fact, at every meal.

I compiled this book of my favorite superfood recipes for my customers originally, proving that superfood can be the star of any meal, even desserts! They have lost weight, improved attitudes, overcome addictions, slowed aging, reduced the effects of osteoporosis and arthritis, and even beat cancer by using these recipes! They are knowledgeable about superfoods, but they have also become superfood geniuses because they have learned how to incorporate their smarts into their everyday lives!

I'm going, being honest, I can't guarantee incredible results, but I can ensure that superfood will give you a natural, no side-effect, kind of improved life and body. There is no superfood diet, but there is a lifestyle of superfood. And I hope this cookbook will be precisely what you need to help make nutritional choices that will significantly impact your life for the decades.

You'll notice the superfoods are bold in every recipe, making it easy for you to see the foods you don't want to replace as you cook. For every meal, there are over 100 delicious and crowd-pleasing recipes in here that you no longer have any excuse not to make superfoods a staple in your diet.

In this food guide, we'll examine the various vegetarian foods you can collect, easily prepare, and add to your long-lasting vegan food stockpile. They are not hard to cook and will satisfy your daily nutritional needs as well as those of your family and loved ones.

Chapter 1: Introducing the Vegetarian Diet

1.1 Defining the Vegetarian Diet

The vegetarian diet is becoming more popular over the past few years. Some studies estimate that more than 18% of the world population is vegetarian.

There are benefits from a well-planned vegetarian diet in several ways. In addition to the economic and ethical benefits of minimizing meat intake, the risk of chronic illness will significantly decrease, weight loss will be increased, and the diet's consistency improved.

This book is a guide to the vegetarian diet for beginners with several delicious and healthy recipes. The traditional vegetarian diet includes poultry, fish, and meat abstinence. Many people follow vegetarian dieting, for ethical purposes, such as animal rights, for personal or religious purposes.

Many choose to become vegetarians for environmental reasons, such as animal production playing a significant role in climate change, rising greenhouse gas emissions, and needing a great deal of electricity, natural resources, and water.

A diet free of meat, fish, and flesh is the basic concept of vegetarianism. Yet vegetarian eating habits include a broad spectrum. Vegetarianism exists in many forms, each with different levels of restriction.

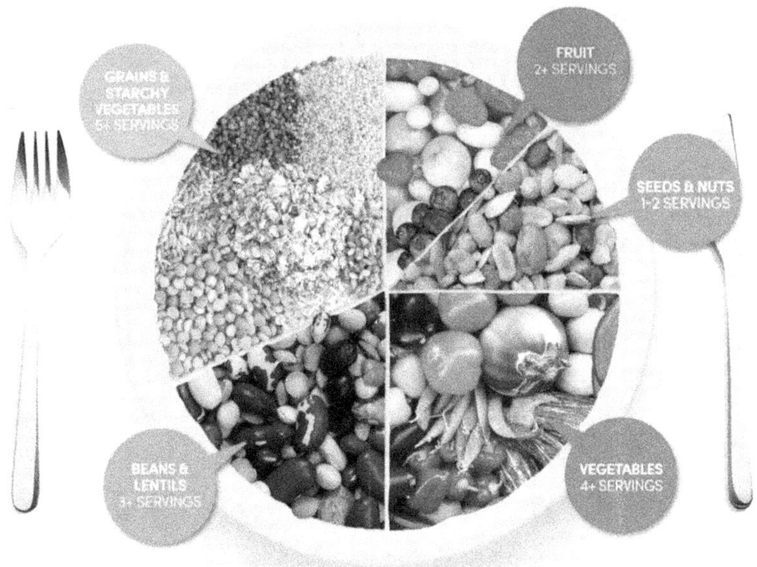

The main types are:

- Lacto-Vegetarian

A lacto-vegetarian consumes milk, but he does not consume any kind of meat or eggs.

- Ovo-Vegetarian Diet

Only eggs are permitted, but dairy products, poultry, fish, and meat are prohibited.

- Lacto-Ovo-Vegetarian Diet:

Water, poultry, and meat are excluded, but milk products and eggs are allowed.

- Pescatarian Diet:

This excludes poultry and meat but requires fish and milk products and eggs in some cases.

- Vegan Diet:

The vegan diet eliminates poultry and meat while allowing fish and milk products and eggs under certain conditions.

- Proletarian:

A vegetarian who eats chicken.

- Pescatarian:

A vegetarian who eats fish.

- Flexitarian Diet:

It is a vegetarian diet with occasional poultry, fish, or meat. Many people who like fruit and veggies over meat are uncomfortable flexitarians.

1.2 Vegetarian Diet Benefits

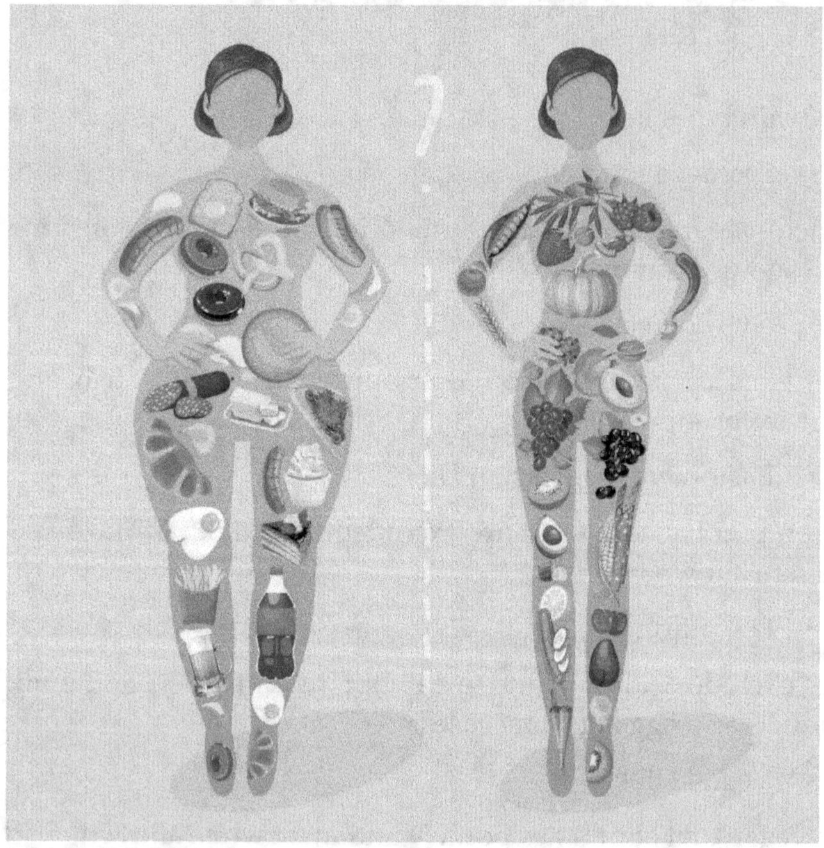

- For Ordinary People

As the gallop survey reveals, an increasing number of people are taking a vegetarian diet. You should do that because:

> It provides safety benefits.
> This is a more environmentally friendly alternative.
> They have concerns about animal treatment.
> They are part of a broader range of lifestyles.

Here are several ways to improve the health of a human by avoiding meat products.

Weight:

Switching to a vegetarian diet can help people lose weight in a 2016 meta-analysis, at least in the short term. To understand how a vegetarian diet can impact weight, scientists need to conduct long-term controlled studies.

Cholesterol:

A systematic analysis conducted in 2015 showed that the average cholesterol level in people who adopt a vegetarian diet is significantly lower.

Cancer:

A study of data by almost 70,000 people has shown that the overall incidence of cancer among vegetarians is lower than in non-vegetarians. The authors suggested that a non-meat diet might provide cancer protection.

Heart Health:

2014 study authors found that people who adopted a vegetarian diet in India were at lower risk for cardiovascular diseases. Studies in western countries had already provided similar findings.

Diabetes:

People who adopt a vegetarian diet can have type 2 diabetes less likely.

Higher consumption of fruits, whole grains, vegetables, legumes and nuts, and a lower intake of unhealthy fats may be essential.

• For Sportsman

Yes, you have heard the same old hoopla all your life: you have to drink a lot of milk and eat plenty of meat to develop strong bones and stay healthy, and nothing else can be more accurate. Yeah, even athletes can succeed on a vegan / plant diet!

There are some advantages of following a plant-based diet compared to one filled with meat and milk from animal mates, and this is not just for you – life with a plant-based diet often helps to decrease global warming, save animal life and plays a significant part in preserving clean air in our climate.

In addition to all the fantastic ways in which your herbal diet can help you save the world, you can also benefit personally. Here are other advantages that you, as a plant-based athlete, will gain from:

Less Clog-Up of the Internal Body

When you eat lots of fruit, vegetables, and whole grains, the food is digested, and the fibers do their job. And all this fiber helps to improve your digestion and reduce bowel flushes, which you can recover from exercise. Leaving the animal products out will also make the veins nice and clean, and you don't have to think about the accumulation and absorption of cholesterol. You can be fast and competitive during competition when you're light and fresh inside.

Great Health Cardiovascular

Since the plant diet is low in cholesterol and saturated fat, you can easily count on cardiovascular health.

The optimal cardiovascular system allows you to run longer, jump higher, and regularly train harder, with quick recovery times between workouts.

If your cardiovascular system works right, it is easier to respire and remain stable and even motivated during your workouts and competitions. So, load up on these carbohydrate and protein-rich menus, such as a sandwich of hummus and avocados, or a tenting chili bowl before you train for the day.

Increased Overall Stamina

Most athletes credit their plant-based diets to greater strength and better sugar in their specific sports. If endurance is essential for any game, from ultimate fighting (think mac Danzig), running races (hears about the precious roll, ever?), its value should not be ignored.

Fortunately, optimum fitness is easy to attain, and a healthy plant-based lifestyle is maintained. The additional stamina makes it easy to manage all activities in life without losing essential time for exercise.

Physical Maintenance Facility

Because plant-based diets don't have saturated fats, maintaining your physique as an athlete is pretty straightforward. If you are running and need to stay lean or want to contend with a muscular but toned body in karate, foods based on plants will help you get there.

Of course, a well-balanced diet is essential – you probably won't have the results to fill up with sucrose snacks and soda. Plenty of grains, legumes, fruits, and veggies are the foundation of every long-term health promotion diet.

The truth is that as a plant-based athlete, there's nothing but advantages. You can rest assured as a reliable, fit vegan that your lifestyle rubs other people who only help reinforce the environment in which we live.

Yeah, and your breath will stay fresh all day long!

Leads to A Quicker Recovery Time

Since whole-food, vegetable-based diets contain a lot of antioxidants, they naturally combat inflammation and oxidative stress (an exercise-induced process that can destroy the cell structure). On the other side, meat includes arachidonic acid, pro-inflammatory fatty acid, cortisol, and c-reactive protein — both dietary bad guys. Instead, fill them with a variety of bright fruits and vegetables, such as leafy greens, sweet potatoes, blueberries, and other rainbow-hued plants.

Boosts Your Strength

Plants are packing an excellent energy boost; just ask former ironman triathlete Brendan brazier, who is now partnering with top athletes to introduce plant-based eating programs. Animal products are bulky and challenging for our bodies to digest and can lead to sluggishness and tiredness. Plants are nutrient-dense, low in fat, and give you more calorie bang for your buck.

Provides A Source of Higher Protein Quality

Although some athletes have long believed that more is better when it comes to protein, it turns out that over-consumption of protein is linked to osteoporosis, kidney disease, calcium stones in the urinary tract, and some cancers. It was also widely believed once that meat was the only source of "complete" protein (containing all nine essential amino acids), but that myth turned out to be nothing more than a bunch of bolognas. Many plants (like quinoa, amaranth, buckwheat, chia seeds, and soya beans, to name a few) have all nine; all the others have six. Either way, if you have a diet of grains, beans, and vegetables, you'll get all the proteins and amino acids you need (and better performance with them).

Provides Fuel

Carbs may often have an unfortunate name, but they're fuel for high-intensity exercise. In athletes, research shows that the availability of carbohydrates improves endurance and efficiency, and whole grains, fruits, and vegetables are good go-to's in carbs. Plus, the plants are high in fiber, so they regulate blood sugar and help sustain you regularly. Since these foods have less fat and are easier to digest, they 're going to help you get quicker, leaner, and more reliable.

According to the physicians' committee for responsible medicine, a healthy diet for athletes serves grains, vegetables, vegetables, and fruit. Combine this magic four, and you're going to hit the ultimate dietary home run. Are you ready to be a big plant? Start the day today!

According to the physicians' committee for responsible medicine, a healthy diet for athletes serves grains, vegetables, vegetables, and fruit. Combine this magic four, and you're going to hit the ultimate dietary home run. Are you ready to be a big plant? Start the day today!

• For the Elderly

A study in 2016 showed that only 1.8% of Americans aged 65 and over adhere to vegetarian diets. Just 2.7 percent of people aged 55 to 64 reported consuming vegetarian foods.

The number of older vegetarians is minimal, and the Preparation arises as to whether a vegetarian diet may be beneficial or detrimental to older adults.

Besides, there are a variety of ways that older adults can benefit from vegetarian diets.

Slow Down Aging

A plant-heavy diet can increase telomeres' activity, which are the reconstructive enzymes found at the end of a cell chromosome.

U.S. Research Department of Defense has found that a plant-based diet can significantly increase the activity of our telomeres, which can help slow down the aging process.

Meanwhile, processed meat was found to have the opposite effect, shortening telomeres over time.

Promote Good Skin

Antioxidants present in plants help to moisturize the skin, repair the tissues of the skin, and eliminate the molecules that cause premature aging.

Recovery of Energy

Energy is linked to digestion. Because it's easier for a senior digestive system to break down plant foods than meat, vegetarian diets can generate more energy throughout the day. And boosting energy is crucial for older adults to get some exercise daily and maintain a happy and healthy lifestyle.

Improving Brain Function

A plant-based diet can help reduce the risk of neurological disorders such as Alzheimer's, and vegetables such as broccoli and cauliflower have properties that can improve brain activity and help you think more clearly.

Lower Stress

A vegetarian diet will lower the levels of cortisol, a stress-related steroid hormone.

Lose Weight

Switching to a vegetarian diet usually means increasing your consumption of fiber and vitamins that promote healthy weight loss.

Sleeping Better

Bananas, sweet potatoes, kale, and nuts are high in vitamin b6, tryptophan, and magnesium. Such essential vitamins and minerals increase melatonin and create a healthy sleep cycle that is especially important for senior health.

1.3 Foods to Be Consumed on A Vegetarian Diet

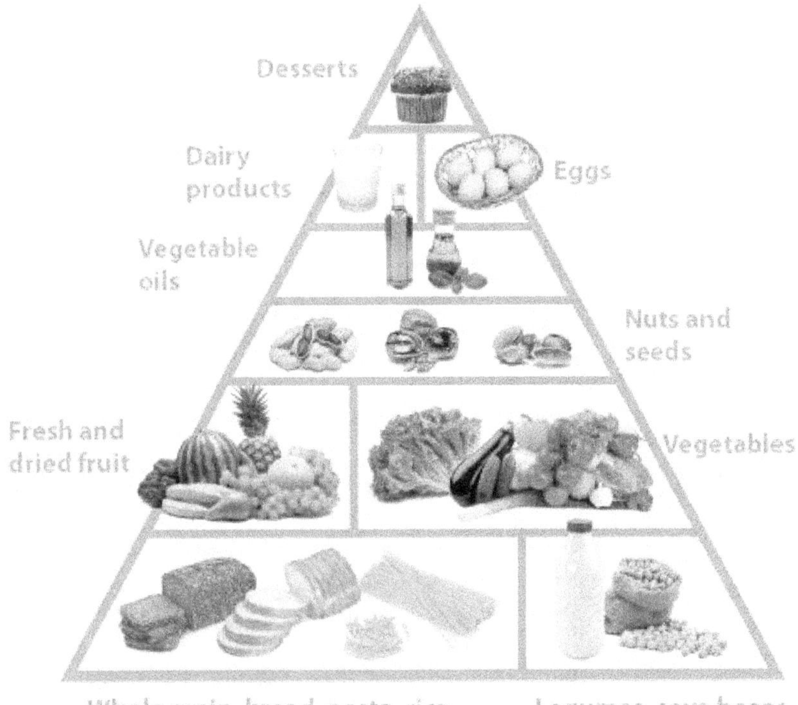

Vegetarian diets should be high in a variety of vegetables, fruits, grains, proteins, and healthy fats.

To complement the meat's protein, add protein-rich plant foods such as seeds, nuts, legumes, tofu, tempeh, and seitan for your diet.

If you follow a lacto-ovo-vegetarian diet, milk and eggs can increase your protein intake.

Stuffing your diet with nutrient-dense whole foods such as vegetables, fruit, and whole grains should improve your body's system with a wide range of essential minerals and vitamins.

Many balanced foods that can be consumed on a vegetarian diet include:

- Protein:

Seitan, tempeh, tofu, milk products, natto, spirulina, eggs, and nutritional yeast.

- Healthy Fat:

Olive oil, coconut oil, avocado

- Seed:

Chia, hemp seeds, and linseeds

- Nuts

Almonds, caskets, chestnuts, and walnuts

- Legumes

Beans, lentils, peas, chickpeas, etc.

- Grains:

Buckwheat, spinach, beans, barley, quinoa

- Vegetable:

Asparagus, leafy greens, tomatoes, carrots, broccoli.

- Fruit:

Berries, bananas, apples, oranges, pears, melons, peaches.

PLANT-BASED vs. VEGAN

	Vegan Diet	Plant-Based Diet	Whole-Food, Plant-Based Diet
Meat & Poultry	No	Avoid	Avoid
Seafood	No	Avoid	Avoid
Eggs & Dairy Products	No	Avoid	Avoid
Oils	OK	OK	Avoid
Highly Processed Foods Refined Sweeteners, Bleached Flours, White Rice	OK	OK	Avoid
Whole Grains Including Whole Grain Flours, Breads, Pastas	OK	OK	OK
Fruits, Veggies, & Starchy Veggies	OK	OK	OK
Legumes	OK	OK	OK

FORKS KNIVES

✓ OK   ~ Avoid   ✗ No

Vegetarianism varies widely, each with its limitations.

The most common vegetarian diet is Lacto-ovo-vegetarian diet. This diet includes the total removal of fish, poultry, and meat.

Individual styles can require the removal of eggs and milk.

The vegan diet is the most restrictive form of vegetarianism. Eggs, fish, poultry, meat, dairy, and other animal foods are entirely barred.

You may have to do away with the following foods depending on what you need and your preferences:

- Meat:

Pork, veal, and beef

- Products for Dairy:

Ovo-vegetarians and vegans must avoid yogurt, milk, and cheese.

- Eggs:

Lacto-vegetarians and vegans must limit their diet's eggs.

- Foods Based on Meat:

Lard, carmine, jelly, oleic acid, suet, and insulated glass.

- Poultry:

Turkish and chicken

- Fish and Shellfish:

Pescatarians are not constrained.

- Other Items for Animals:

Vegans will limit their diet to beeswax, pollen, and honey.

1.5 Best Vegetarian Foods in Term of Macros

What Are Macros?

Macro is a term for macronutrients abbreviated. Macronutrients are essential nutrients that we use to function in large quantities, rather than small amounts of micronutrients. The three macronutrients that we need are carbohydrates, fats, and protein that we get through feeding.

EASY VEGAN MACROS

CARBS

- energy source
- blood glucose regulation

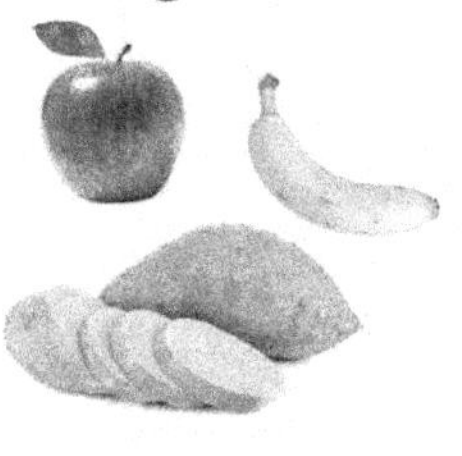

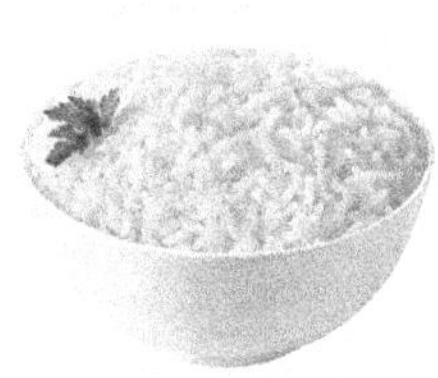

PROTEIN

- builds & repairs muscle tissue
- essential amino acids
- regulate activities of cells & organs

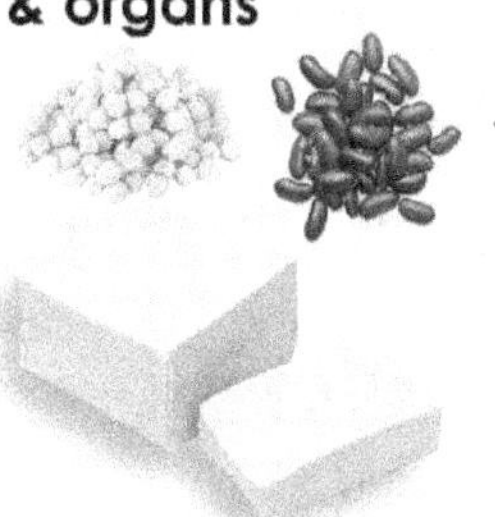

FAT

- insulates body
- esential fatty acids (omega 3's)
- regulates hormone production

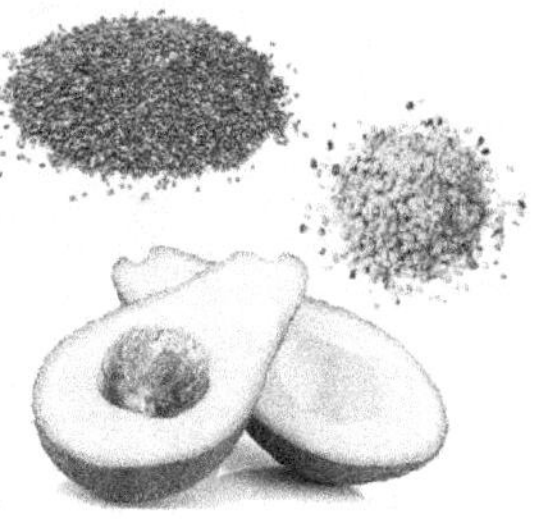

In the form of macros, below are some of the best vegetarian foods:

- Oil MCT

I love MCT oil in my diet as a source of fat. I want to add 1 tsp of it in my pre-training coffee in the morning to get my daily rock! Coconut and olive are other oils I use.

- Banana

You can consume one of the simplest, most compact, and flexible, nutrient-dense, fat-free carbohydrate types. Moreover, they are always a lovely, sweet treat. At least one I eat every day. Try these ten banana snacks and desserts ideas. You do have to try my flourless banana protein brownies!

- Tempeh

I typically eat tempeh 3-4 times a week. I haven't had much of it before, but it's such a good source of protein in a vegan diet that I've added to my weekly tofu routine. Although the calories are a little higher, tempeh is less than tofu, and it is generally healthier because it contains more protein and fiber. You will find it in most organic foods or well-stocked grocery stores if you never tried tempeh. Toss it into your recipes and add it to soups, salads, casseroles, or pasta sauces. Tempah adds chewy consistency and extra protein and fiber to your dishes.

I also like marinated tempeh cooked or dry-fry to be extra crispy and add the strips into salads or sandwiches.

- Cauliflower Rice

A low-calorie, low-carbon, healthy, and delicious rice alternative. Just a cauliflower head big and use it everywhere your rice!

- Powdered Peanut Butter

Without powdered peanut butter, I'm not sure I might stick to macros. Powdered peanut butter can be combined with water to spread low fat or in some foods, oats, smoothies, and sauces. A serving of powdered peanut butter has just 45 calories, which makes a perfect substitute for those who enjoy peanut butter though it's certainly not the real thing! I love both standard peanut butter powdered and chocolate!

- Protein Powders (Plant-Based)

Protein powder, therefore. I cannot get the amount of protein that I want without, anyway, without eating a lot of carbohydrates and fat. I do my utmost to stick to the cleanest protein supplements based on most foods I can find. This means that I use plenty of organic brown rice protein, natural hemp protein, and several other plant-based products.

- Squash, Yams and Potatoes Sweet

Magnificent, clean, safe, rich in vitamins, pure carbohydrates. My favorite way to use potatoes and sweet potatoes are to make fried oven without oil. Simply wedge your potato, season, and bake to crispy. I will recommend boiling potato or sweet potato for a few minutes before baking. I like baked sweet potatoes, and I usually throw some in the oven on Sundays, so that they're ready for the week. You just don't have to add anything because they're so good single! Sweet potato breakfast bowls are also amazing!

- Nutritional Yeast

I love nutritional yeast as it has a fragrance, and it contains b vitamins. Nutritional yeast is a complete protein, which means that it includes the nine essential acids that your body can not produce from the 18 amino acids.

Nutritional yeast also produces beta-1, 3-glucan, trehalose, mannan, and glutathione compounds that are associated with increased immunity, reduced cholesterol rates, and prevention of cancer. A large dosage of iron, selenium, and zinc minerals is also provided when you eat nutritional yeast. I apply it to pasta, smoothies, cookies, sprinkle on salads, and make sauces.

- Raw Vegetables

You 're going to want to store up on all the raw veggies you can get on. It's your best bet to build filling yet low-calorie foods that suit your macros. At least one big salad I eat a day, and it not only fills me but at the same time, I have a ton of micronutrients. I would especially suggest concentrating on the dark leafy greens for the micronutrients they contain! After that, eat the rainbow, and you're all set!

- Mustard Dijon

Dijon mustard is my favorite condiment for low-calorie, fatty, spicy sauces, and clothing.

- Spirulina

Spirulina is one of the most nutritious sources of food on the planet and is noted for its highest protein content by weight. Moreover, the protein it contains is highly digestible, bioavailable, and "full," which means that it includes all the essential amino acids.

This also provides a wide variety of vitamins, phytonutrients, and antioxidants, which has been shown to improve recovery from stress further. I usually add this to my morning smoothie; it doesn't taste great so that you wouldn't drink something. I sometimes apply it to a big glass of lemon water, but it's usually adequate to mask the flavor. I do use chlorella; you can see it as an alternative. They are also available as powder or capsules.

- Seeds Hemp

Strong in protein and healthy fats such as omega-3 and low in carbohydrates, hemp seeds must be a dietary necessity of vegan life. I typically have 1-2 tbsp to my morning oats, but you can also add smoothies, sprinkle on salads, add desserts, and just take a spoon to it!

- Oats

High in fiber and vitamins, energy, low fat, and delicious carbohydrates to fuel and maintain your workouts. I eat one serving of 1/2 cup of oats per day, and every time I look forward to them!

On Sundays, I prepare overnight oats for a week. I'll just slice my oats, chia seeds, hemp seeds, and other additions into five containers and throw it into the cupboard the night before I'm going to eat it. I only take out every night and top it with almond milk and put it in the fridge for a good, fresh, delicious breakfast.

Get some meal prep containers for yourself!

- Tofu (Organic)

Get enough protein while keeping your carbohydrates and fat under control would be your biggest challenge with a balanced diet on plants. Many higher protein vegetable foods also contain high carbohydrates. Tofu is well balanced, and you'd find it hard to get through at least a couple of times a week without eating. You can add additional firm tofu to your delicious dishes or make perfect vegan ricotta, or use soft tofu for tasty, high-protein vegan desserts. I suggest that you store a few blocks every week.

- Lentils

Since they take a while to cook, I want to prepare a large batch of lentils during the weekend to add protein to my meals all week long. Lenses provide about 9 g of protein for 116 calories and virtually no fat, making it a perfect addition to a diet focused on plants.

The lens is also fiber-high and has vast quantities of micronutrients such as magnesium, folate, and iron. They can be used in a wide variety of dishes and are also inexpensive.

- Spices, Onion, And Garlic Herbs

Keep your food savory and tasty, and give a range of loads of different herbs and spices, reducing the amount of salt you need. I always add onion and garlic to almost all, are rich in antioxidants of all kinds, and are a perfect addition to any diet.

- Sriracha, Salsa, Other Sauces

Again, spice up your dishes with the low-fat options!

- Drops (Organic Stevia)

Using as a sweetener, I used to use a lot of maple syrup but add some teaspoons, and the carbs would go off before you know it. I cut out the maple syrup and turn as a sweetener to organic stevia drops, I just wear it a little here and there, generally if I want a sweet evening treat, but want my macro objectives to continue during the day. That said, you have to eat more carbohydrates by the end of the day, sure, hit the syrup!

- Berries

Berries are highly nutrient-dense and, as far as fruit goes, relatively low carbohydrate. I eat one serving of mixed berries every day for the benefit of the micronutrient and the delicious sweet treat! I like to add them to my morning oats, or even make a dessert in the evenings.

- Vinegar

I like to keep my pantry stocked with a variety of vinegar to make dressings and sauces. It's a great way to add a ton of flavor without adding any extra macros to your day. My favorite is apple cider vinegar, balsamic vinegar, rice vinegar, and white wine vinegar. I use them in homemade salad dressings every day.

- Edamame

Edamame is a wonderful high-protein, low-carbon food that you can enjoy on your own or add to all sorts of dishes. I like to make a lot of Sundays to enjoy all week long.

- Water

Don't forget to be hydrated all day long! It's always a good idea to drink a large glass in the morning as well as before going to bed. In the morning, I like to add apple cider vinegar to my water to help me alkalize my body and start digestion.

Chapter 2: Vegetarian Meal Prepping

2.1 Getting Started with Vegetarian Meal Prepping

Sure, nutritious, home-made vegetarian food is within your grasp — and within your cooking capacity. — but if you don't have the supplies, you can't cook. What do you need to do? Yeah, what you're expected to store up depends on your particular circumstances. Do you live in a dorm with a shared kitchen that provides students with pots, pans, and other necessary cooking options? Are you staying in an off-campus apartment? No matter the case, most of the basics are inexpensive and can typically be purchased in discount stores — and a few simple items are going a long way.

- Kitchen Supplies

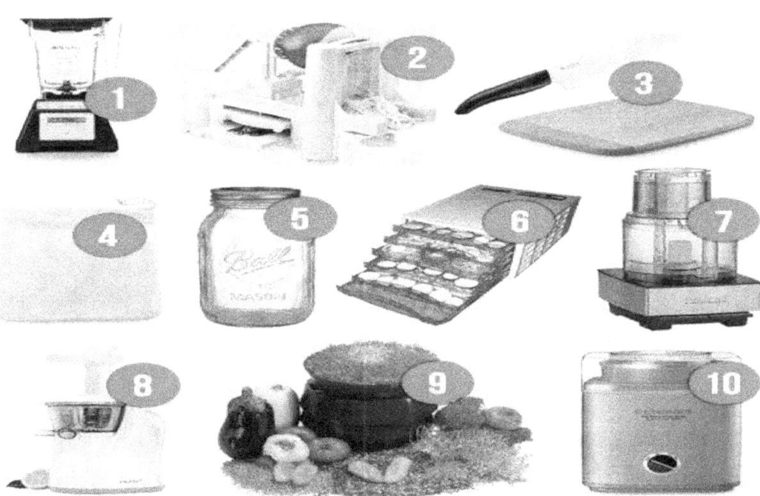

To continue with, you want to make sure you have the kitchen supplies you need to make vegetarian and vegan dishes that you love.

You can buy a lot of these cheap supplies, and it's much better to buy them all in advance than to run out late at night when you just have to have mini goat cheese pizzas or no-bake cocoa balls. So, to prevent any kind of food emergency, make sure you have the following on hand:

- Cleaver (knife)
- Refrigerator
- Heat-proof rubber spatula
- Measurement of spoons and measuring cup
- Colander of metal
- Plastic mixing bowls for mixing Ingredients and serving dishes
- Peeler of vegetables
- Whiskey
- Wood or bamboo cutting board
- Wood or bamboo spoon
- Zester's

Besides, if there is space in your budget — and your dorm or student residence permits — there are some simple electrical appliances that could come in handy:

- Coffee maker
- Hot plate or rice cooker
- Microwave oven
- Food processor
- Toaster or toaster oven

Once you have purchased the necessary cooking tools, you may want to buy your food portioning containers. This way, one recipe is going to give you multiple meals. A little time in the kitchen could feed you all week long — and, with all the time you spend cramming for exams and hanging out with your friends, anything that can save you time in the kitchen is perfect.

- Stock the Pantry

You'll need to read through each recipe before deciding what fresh Ingredients you need to buy, but that doesn't mean that you can't store your pantry with dry parts and some canned food for quick meals. Try loading on the following vegetarian essentials:

Goods for Baking

- All-purpose flour
- Sugar (raw)
- Unsweetened cocoa powder
- Whole-grain flour

Beans (Canned or Dry)

- Adzuki black
- Butter
- Cannellini's
- Chickpeas
- Dried lentils
- Kidney
- Pinto
- Black-eyed peas

Dry Herbs and Spices

- Basil
- Leaf of The Bay
- Pepper from Cayenne
- Cinnamon
- Coriander
- Cumin
- Curry
- Fresh Ground Pepper
- Powder of Garlic
- Ginger
- Nutritional Yeast
- The Oregano
- Parsley

- Rosemary
- Sea Salt
- Whole-Wheat Pasta

Flavors

- Apple vinegar
- Balsamic vinegar
- Dijon mustard
- Rice vinegar
- Soya sauce or tamari
- Tomato sauce
- Honey
- Lemon juice

Grains

- Brown rice
- Buckwheat
- Quinoa
- Oats (rolled)
- Berries of wheat

Oils

- Coconut oil
- Peanut oil
- Sesame oil
- Olive oil

When you've got the basics, you 're good to start cooking! So, say goodbye to peanut butter and jelly sandwiches and pasta from the dining room and hello to delicious vegetarian meals that fill you up without emptying your wallet!

2.2 Equipment Required for The Preparation of Meals

Honestly, you can make your meal prepping work with only the most straightforward kitchen equipment, much of which you probably already have at home.

But to give you an idea of how to streamline your meal prep session, we want to provide you with a quick overview of the best tools.

- Basic Cooking Tools

Whether you want to follow our meal plan or just step up your home cooking game, there are a few devices that we suggest you have on hand that will make preparing nutritious and delicious meals a breeze.

- Blender
- Parchment paper or silicone mats
- Cutting board
- Non-stick pan
- Food processor
- Knives
- Baking sheets
- Instant Pot (for safe hands-off batch cooking; perfect for grains, legumes and stews)

The last three items are more of a "nice-to-have," and you can still make our meal plan or plant-based eating work without them.

- Food-Storage Equipment

- Plastic food containers or Tupperware
- Glass jars and boxes
- Bento-style boxes or lunch boxes
- Ziplock-style food bags

2.3 Tips for Cooking A Range of Ready-To-Go Meals in One Day

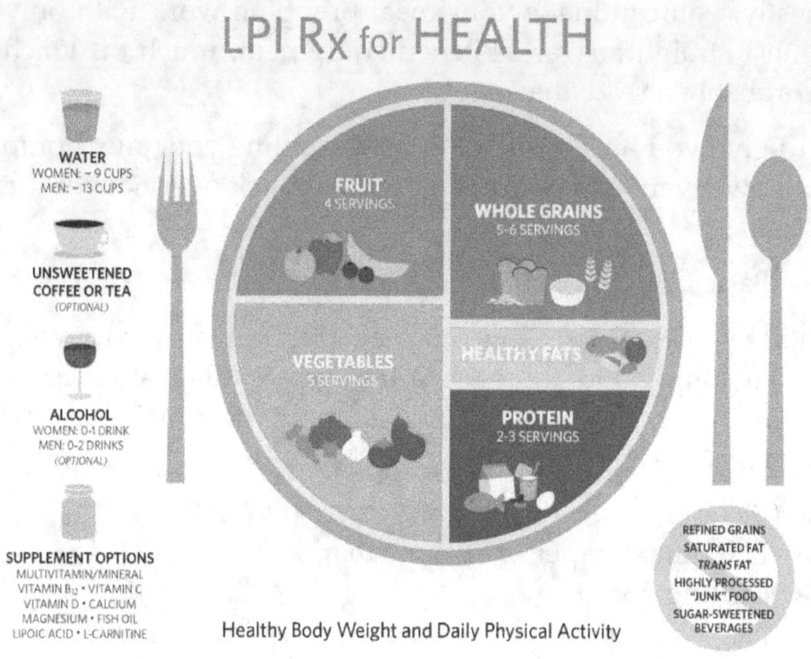

As a vegetarian, I'm sure you 're already familiar with getting the right nutrition from non-meat sources. Setting up for emergencies requires a similar degree of savviness, but with a little more energy since fresh fruits and vegetables have a limited shelf life. Foods that you intend to pack into your emergency food kit will not need refrigeration, very little or no cooking preparation, and little to no water. You should include at least one gallon of water per person per day in your kit, so it's okay to store some food that needs water to be prepared. These few tips are going to make sure you 're

Have a sufficient quantity of vegetarian food at hand, beginning with proper storage techniques.

- Adequate Storage

Buy food that has a long shelf life when you get to the grocery store. Buy in bulk and store in an air-tight storage container. You can also store food storage containers free of BPA. Putting the silica packets inside the box will prevent problems related to the container from occurring.

- Humidity

Ensure that all food containers are washed with soap and water before transport. Store the food containers in your pantry and never pack them too high, especially if you stay in an area that is prone to natural disasters. Choose a cool, dark, and dry spot with a minimum temperature of 32 degrees and not more than 70 degrees Fahrenheit.

- Canned Food

Even vegetarians will not eat canned food in usual circumstances. Yet when you're faced with an emergency, the story is different. The comfort they offer is going to make you grateful. You can eat most of the canned food right out of the can. They do not need any special preparation, water, or cooking. Purchase fruit, tomatoes, beans, fish, milk, pasta, and sardines. It is better and healthier to buy low-sugar or low-sodium products such as fruit in light syrup with no added sugar. They 're more costly, but they're 100% expensive.

- Protein

As a vegetarian, you 're not a meat-eater, but you're talking about having nutrition from non-animal sources. It's worth understanding that certain protein products have a shallow shelf life. Emergency food choices include lentils, beans, rice, milk (all canned), nut butter, seeds, nuts, and meat-free or vegan suckers.

Protein powder is another excellent option and can be stored easily.

You may blend protein powder into a healthy pudding or add canned juice and water to make a tasty, nutritious drink. People with dietary restrictions can do with rice-based, gluten-free, and lactose-free protein powders. They are readily available. A serving of tuna or beans with two protein shakes can provide enough protein for a day.

- Freeze-Dried Food

Freeze-dried products are available in several bulk sizes. And you should know that individual mylar freeze-dried fruit pouches have a shelf life of up to two decades. You may enjoy them as a snack or combine them with healthy staple foods such as caramel sauces, pasta, cereals, and apple sauce to improve the nutritional, caloric, and taste.

Vegetables are sold in different sizes, with a shelf life of up to 25 years.

2.4 Tips for Food Preservation

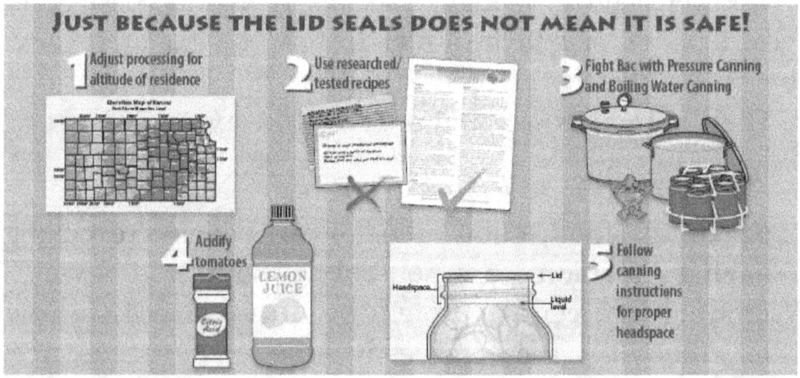

- Best-Stored Foods on The Counter

Cucumber:

Keep them out of the refrigerator. Put them on your kitchen counter instead.

Onion:

You can place onions on the table, but you can't get close to the potatoes. Cut onions are to be processed in the refrigerator.

Tomato:

Tomatoes are best stored in a spacious, airy setting, so the kitchen counter is the best! Yet try not to stack them on top of each other. Keep them a few inches away from each other.

Asparagus:

Cut the lower-inch stalks and put them in a bowl of water to keep them fresh.

Basil:

Apply the same technique to basil asparagus. It will preserve their flavor and freshness for days to come.

Certain Vegetables and Fruits That You Can Store on The Counter Include:

Bananas, bananas, mangoes, papaya, grapes, ginger, eggplant, pineapple, lemons, watermelon, lime, and pomegranate.

- Foods Best Stored in The Dark

Potatoes:

Place in a cool, dry spot. I will suggest a kitchen cabinet.

Garlic:

Garlic is best kept in the dark. Place it in a paper bag to keep it fresh for weeks.

Other vegetables and fruits that can be kept in the dark include:

Butternut squash, acorn squash, spaghetti squash, banana squash, Spring carrots, sweet potatoes.

- The Food Best Stored in The Fridge

Parsley and Cilantro:

Take the bottom inch of the stems and placed the vegetables in a bowl of water. They 're going to last up to five days in the refrigerator.

Vegetables such as broccoli and bell peppers last long in wet weather, so you can store them in a refrigerator while regulating the humidity.

Fruits such as grapes and blueberries are best kept in dry areas. Just hold them together in a drawer where the humidity turned low. It would keep them healthy for more extended periods.

Certain Vegetables and Fruits That You Can Keep in The Refrigerator Include:

Carrots, peas, radishes, corn, broccoli, cauliflower, green onion, lettuce, okra, mushrooms, artichokes, beets, leafy vegetables, like beans, Brussels, celery, leeks, spinach, zucchini, yellow squash, green beans.

Remove the Following Foods from The Counter and Place Them in The Refrigerator:

Plums, kiwis, pears, peaches, avocados, nectarines.

Chapter 3: Healthy Vegetarian Breakfast, Lunch and Dinner Recipes

3.1 Breakfast -Sweet and Salty Recipes

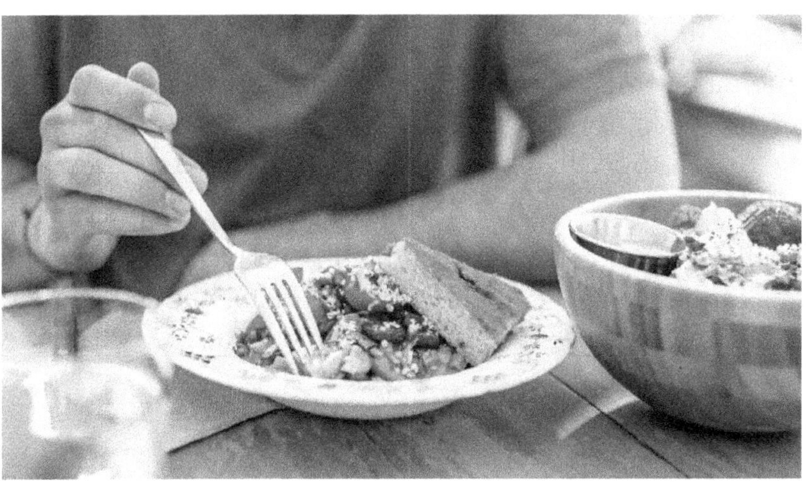

Dried Blueberry and Hempseed Muffins

Ingredients

- ✓ One-fourth of a cup of wheat bran
- ✓ Take 1 1/4 cup wheat flour
- ✓ Flaxseed meal 2 tablespoons
- ✓ 1 and 1/2 baked soda teaspoons
- ✓ 1 1/2 teaspoons ground cinnamon
- ✓ One teaspoons bakery powder
- ✓ 1/2 teaspoon salt
- ✓ 2/3 cup dark brown sugar packed
- ✓ 2/3 of a cup of dried blueberries
- ✓ 1/2 cup of hemp seeds
- ✓ 3 Tablespoons of vegetable oil
- ✓ 1 and 1/3 cups of simple soy yogurt
- ✓ 1 big, ripe, peeled and sliced banana
- ✓ 2-3 handfuls of fresh, chopped spinach

Directions

1. Preheat the oven to 400 ° f. Using a 12-cup muffin box with paper liners.

2. Mix the bran, flour, flaxseeds, bakery powder, soda, cinnamon, salt, and brown sugar in a large bowl. Stir in the superfood, dried wheat, and hemp seeds. Then mix them.

3. Combine oil, yogurt, banana, and spinach in a blender. Blend at average speed until the mixture is smooth. In the large bowl, put the mixed Ingredients over the dry Ingredients. Stir gently until all Ingredients are moisturized.

4. Spoon the batter carefully into the lined muffin tin. Bake the muffins for between 18 and 20 minutes. Enable the cupcakes to cool a few minutes before they are removed and transferred to a cooling wire rack.

Yield: 12 muffins

2. Sandwich Zucchini Bagel

Gluten free

Prep: 25 min Cook: 17 min makes four bagels

Ingredients

- ✓ Cooking spray non-stick
- ✓ 3 cups grated zucchini
- ✓ 1 cup of mozzarella cheese shredded
- ✓ 1/3 cup of coconut flour.
- ✓ One teaspoon bakery powder
- ✓ 1/4 teaspoon is salt.
- ✓ 2 big eggs
- ✓ 1 cup of white egg
- ✓ One teaspoon hot sauce.

Directions

1. Preheat the oven to 400 degrees f. Spray the cooking spray on a donut model.

2. Put the grated zucchini in the sink and let it drain for 20 minutes. Transfer to a cheesecloth or several towels and squeeze out all excess humidity. The zucchini should be slightly dry.

3. Heat the mozzarella cheese in a small microwave bowl until it melts in 30 seconds

4. Mix the cocoa flour, drained zucchini, baking powder, salt, and whole eggs in a large bowl.

5. Add the melted mozzarella and mix until a dough is formed with your clean hands. Divide the batter evenly between 4 cavities of the mold.

6. Bake until bagels are set with no sign of jiggling 15 to 17 minutes. Remove and cool. Detach. Turn the pot upside down and shake to put the bagels on a plate. Place aside. Set aside.

7. Over medium heat, heat a medium non-stick skillet.

8. Add the white egg and cook, without stirring, for 3 to 4 minutes or until no longer bright and runny. Cover the eggs and turn them in half. Cook for another 1 minute. Remove the eggs from the saucepan and cut it into four squares. Drizzle with hot sauce each piece lightly. Set aside to cool.

9. In each of 4 serving 24-ounce meal prepare containers or quarter-size resealable bags, place one bagel and one egg white square. Hot for up to 5 days.

Reheat:

Reheat the bagel 20-30 seconds in the microwave with the egg white. This heat quickly!

Freeze:

Freeze any remaining dough for up to 1 month in a quarterly resealable freezer bag—Thaw in the refrigerator after the Directions for the recipe overnight before cooking.

The finished bagel sandwiches can also be freeze for up to 1 month.

Per serving (1 bagel and white egg): fat: 10 g; protein: 21 g; total carbohydrate: 20 g; net carbohydrate: 10 g; fiber: 10 g; sugar: 2 g; sodium: 418 mg.

3. Muffins of Pecan and Zucchini

Ingredients

- ✓ 1 1/3 cups of wheat flour
- ✓ 2/3 cup bran
- ✓ Baking powder 2 teaspoons
- ✓ One teaspoon of cinnamon ground
- ✓ 3⁄4 teaspoons of salt
- ✓ 1⁄4 teaspoon ground cloves
- ✓ Two-thirds of cup granulated sugar
- ✓ 2 Big bananas, mashed
- ✓ 1/3 cup of vegetable oil
- ✓ ¼ cup of hemp or coconut milk
- ✓ One teaspoon extract of vanilla
- ✓ 2 cups zucchini, coarsely shredded and not peeled (more nutrients!)
- ✓ 1⁄2 cup of pecans, sliced

Directions

1. Preheat the oven to 375 ° f. Prepare your 12-muffin tin with fat or fill each cup with liners of paper.

2. In a large bowl, whisk the flour, bran, baking powder, cinnamon, salt, and cloves. Combine sugar, bananas, butter, milk, and coffee in another smaller pot. Blend the Ingredients until all is well balanced and frothy. Attach the zucchini and mix water.

3. Combine the wet mix with the dry mixture and blend until blended. Remove the pecans by folding them gently.

4. Place the batter into the muffin cups evenly. Bake for about 28 minutes or until a toothpick gets clean. Enable the muffins to refresh for a few minutes in the tin before moving to a cooling wire rack.

Yield: 12 muffins

4. Muffins with Cranberries and Orange

Ingredients

- ✓ 2/3 cup of dried cranberries, unsweetened
- ✓ 1/2 cup of hot water
- ✓ 1 tablespoon agave nectar
- ✓ Take 1 cup of wheat flour.
- ✓ 1 cup of white flour unbleached
- ✓ One tablespoon flaxseed, ground;
- ✓ 3/4 cup of sugar.
- ✓ One small banana, mashed
- ✓ One teaspoon bakery powder
- ✓ One teaspoon of baking soda
- ✓ 1/2 teaspoon salt.
- ✓ 1/2 cup of orange juice
- ✓ 1/2 cup of coconut milk
- ✓ 1/3 tablespoon apple sauce, unsweetened
- ✓ One teaspoon vanilla
- ✓ One teaspoon orange zest grated

Directions

1. Add cranberries in a bowl and pour hot water and agave nectar on top. Lift all together and leave the cranberries to stand before they continue to plump for 15 to 20 minutes.

2. Preheat the oven to 400 degrees f, and line with the paper pad a two 12-cup muffin tin. This recipe will yield around 14 to 16 muffins.

3. Combine flours, flaxseeds, sugar, mashed banana, bakery powder, soda, and salt in a large bowl. Mix the orange juice, chocolate butter, applesauce, vanilla, and orange zest in a separate dish. Using a filter to extract the cranberries from the liquid and then dump the fluid in the other fluid mix.

4. Use your fingers in the middle of the dry Ingredients to make a well. Put the liquid mix into the center. Use a wooden spoon to combine all the Ingredients, so that the meal is not over-moistened. Add the cranberries then.

5. Use a spoon to divide the batter between the muffin cups evenly. Put 12 to 15 minutes in the oven or until the toothpick is pure when inserted into a muffin core.

6. Enable the muffins to cool for at least 5 minutes before being removed from the tin and put on the wire refrigerator.

Return: 14 to 16 muffins

5. Cinnamon Streusel Muffins Blueberry

Ingredients

- ✓ 1 cup of almond or cocoa milk
- ✓ Take 1 tablespoon of apple vinegar cider
- ✓ 1/4 of a cup of field flaxseed
- ✓ Take 1 cup of wheat meal
- ✓ 3/4 cup of all-purpose meal
- ✓ 1 1/2 baked soda teaspoons.
- ✓ 1 teaspoon of cinnamon ground
- ✓ 1/4 teaspoon conventional oil.
- ✓ 1/4 cup of olive oil extra virgin.
- ✓ 1/2 cup of pure maple syrup.
- ✓ 1 tablespoon pure extract of vanilla.
- ✓ 1/2 teaspoon pure extract of almond.
- ✓ Approximately 1 1/2 cup fresh blueberries

For the Streusel Cinnamon:

- ✓ 2 tablespoons plus two turbinado sugar teaspoons.

- ✓ One tablespoon of cinnamon.
- ✓ Healthy vegan butter
- ✓ 2 teaspoons flour
- ✓ A salt pinches

Directions

1. Preheat the oven to 375 ° f. By filling it with paper liners, prepare a 12-cup muffin tray.

2. In a small cup, mix vinegar and milk and set aside. In a medium bowl, mix all the dry Ingredients and whisk together. Combine all the wet Ingredients in another smaller pot.

3. Then add the wet Ingredients to the dry Ingredients, mix. Cut the blueberries.

4. Prepare the cinnamon streusel top by mixing it in a small bowl with all the Ingredients.

5. Spread the batter uniformly into the muffin cups. Until baking, sprinkle with the strip top for 15 to 20 minutes or until golden and robust. Allow the muffins to cool for almost 15 minutes or more before serving.

Yield: 12 muffins

6. Vegetarian micas

Nut free

Prep: 5 min. Cook: 7 min. Serving 3

Ingredients

- ✓ Nonstick cooking spray
- ✓ 3 Cups of egg whites
- ✓ 1/2 teaspoon ground cumin.
- ✓ 6 corn tortillas (yellow or white), cut in pieces in bite size
- ✓ Cotija cheese, six pieces, crumbled.
- ✓ Six tablespoons of lime salsa.
- ✓ Six tablespoons Pico de Gallo or store-bought Pico

Directions

1. Over medium-high cook heat a large skillet. Coat the saucepan with water.

2. Add the whites of egg, cumin, and tortillas. Cook with a spatula for 1 to 2 minutes until the eggs are finished.

3. Add cheese and cook, stirring, for another 1 minute, or until the eggs are shiny.

4. Divide the egg mixture equally between the three 24-once single-serve preparation containers and let it cool before sealing. In each of the 3 (2-ounce) lid cups and two tablespoons of Pico de Gallo in each of the 3 (2-ounce) lid additional cups, placed two tablespoons of green salsa. Cool the containers up to 5 days.

Reheat:

In the microwave, heat the egg whites in 30 seconds until the desired temperature is reached.

Per serving (1 egg white container with greens and Gallo peaks): calories: 315; fat: 6 g; Protein: 33 g.; totals: 31 g. Carbs; net carbs: 28 g. Fiber: 3 g.

7. Pudding Overnight Tropical Chia

(free-gluten, no cook)

Prep: 10 minutes, plus 4 hours or more to prepare Serves 5

Ingredients

- ✓ 21/2 cups of unsweetened almond milk
- ✓ 21/2 scoops of almond (whey or vegan) protein powder
- ✓ Divided into 1 cup of fresh pineapple plus 5 tablespoons
- ✓ Seeds of chia 3/4 cup
- ✓ 1 tablespoon maple syrup
- ✓ Extract of coconut 21/4 teaspoons
- ✓ 5 tablespoons of unsweetened flakes of coconut

Directions

1. Whisk up the sugar, protein powder, 1 cup of pineapple, chia seeds, maple syrup, and coconut extract in a big bowl until mixed. Divide the pudding into 5 Mason jars (8-ounce) with lids.

2. Add one tablespoon of coconut flakes and 1 tablespoon of the remaining pineapple to each jar. If you want the coconut flakes to stay crunchy, break them into five resealable snack-size packets.

3. Seal the reeds. Refrigerate overnight, or at least for 4 hours, and the pudding can dry. The pudding is kept for up to 5 days, refrigerated.

Calories: 375; fat: 22 g; protein: 17 g; total carbohydrates: 28 g; net carbohydrates: 12 g; fiber: 16 g; sugar: 7 g; sodium: 231 mg

8. Coconut Greek Pancakes Yogurt

Prep: 7 min. Cook: 10 min. Serves 2

Ingredients

- ✓ Six large white eggs
- ✓ 1 cup of dried oats
- ✓ 3⁄4 cup of oat flour
- ✓ Vanilla protein powder (whey or vegan) 3 tablespoons
- ✓ 1 Bananas
- ✓ 3⁄4 cup plain Greek yogurt
- ✓ Baking soda 3⁄4 tablespoon
- ✓ 2 tablespoons unsweetened coconut flakes, plus more topping
- ✓ Extract 1⁄4 tablespoon of coconut
- ✓ 5 drops liquid Stevia (optional)
- ✓ Non-stick spray
- ✓ 1 cup raspberries

Directions

1. At medium-high pressure, preheat a griddle or large skillet.

2. Combine the egg whites, oats, oat flour, protein powder, banana, yogurt, baking soda, coconut flakes, coconut extract, and liquid stevia (if used) in a high-power blender. Blend in for about 1 minute at high speed. The batter will be somewhat thinner than a regular pancake batter.

3. Coat the skillet with spray to fry. In a palm, scale circle applies about 1/3 cup of the batter to the skillet. Cook it for 1 to 2 minutes, turn over, and cook for another 1 to 2 minutes, until light gray. Set aside to freshen up. Repeat with the remaining batter, retrieving the pan as necessary.

4. Put three pancakes into each of the resealable two quarter size bags. Put 1/2 cup of berries in each of 2 resealable sandwich or snack shaped containers. Refrigerate for five days.

Heat:

In the microwave, heat the pancakes for 30 to 45 seconds.

Freeze:

Those are freezing well. Place the pancakes in a resealable, gallon-sized freezer bag, stacked flat between each pancake with wax paper or parchment to prevent sticking. Freeze till one month — thaw overnight at the refrigerator.

Calories: 714; fat: 17 g; protein: 60 g; total carbohydrate: 81 g; net carbohydrate: 66 g; fiber: 15 g; sugar: 17 g; sodium: 644 mg;

9. Superfood Shake

Gluten-free dairy free, no cook, vegan

Prep: 5 minutes serves 1

Ingredients

- ✓ 1 Banana
- ✓ 1/2 cup of whole or cut fresh strawberries

- ✓ 1/2 cups of kale cut washed and dried.
- ✓ 1/2 cup spinach
- ✓ 1 spoonful of coconut oil, cashew butter or almond butter
- ✓ 1 cup of almond unsweetened milk
- ✓ 1 scoop vegan vanilla protein powder

Directions

1. Combine the pineapple, tomatoes, broccoli, spinach, and coconut oil in a quarter shaped freezer container. Freeze till one month.

2. When making the shake, combine the contents of the freezer bag, almond milk, and protein powder in a high-power blender. Mix for almost 1 minute on high speed, until smooth.

Per serving (1 shake): Calories: 386; Fat: 21g; Protein: 24g; Total carbs: 43g; Net carbs: 33g; Fiber: 10g; Sugar: 18g; Sodium: 430mg

10. Sweet Potato Breakfast Burritos

Nut-free

Prep: 15 min. Cook: 20 min. Serves 8

Ingredients

- ✓ 1 tablespoon of olive oil
- ✓ Chopped 1/2 golden onion
- ✓ 2 Cloves of garlic, minced
- ✓ 2 cups cubed sweet potato
- ✓ One red bell pepper, chopped
- ✓ One and a half teaspoons of smoked paprika
- ✓ ½ teaspoon salt, plus more for seasoning
- ✓ ½ teaspoon freshly ground black pepper, plus more for seasoning
- ✓ 3 cups egg whites
- ✓ Non-stick spray

✓ 4 Cut Da Carb wraps, or other low-carb wraps, halved horizontally
✓ 8 (3/4-ounce) spreadable cheese wedges
✓ 2 cups canned reduced-sodium black beans, drained and rinsed
✓ 1 cup of Greek non-fat yogurt
✓ 1 salsa cup

Directions

1. Heat the olive oil in a big skillet on normal heat, until it shines.

2. Add the onion and cook for 2 to 3 minutes, until slightly softened.

3. Pour in the garlic, sweet potato, red pepper bell, paprika, salt, and pepper. Remove to combine, reduce heat to medium-low, cover the skillet, and cook for 8 minutes or tender until the sweet potato. Uncover the skillet and simmer for another 5 minutes, stirring regularly until the excess moisture evaporates, and the sweet potatoes on the edges are soft, caramelized, and crispy. Set aside.

4. In a large bowl, whisk the egg whites.

5. Put another medium skillet over medium heat and coat it with cooking spray. Pour the eggs into the skillet and cook for 2 minutes, continually stirring with a spatula, until the eggs are just cooked. Transfer the eggs to a medium bowl and set aside.

6. Put the wraps on a work surface. Spread one wedge of cheese down the center of each cover. Add ¼ cup of scrambled egg whites, ¼ cup of black beans, and ¼ cup of sweet potato hash to the center of each wrap. Fold and wrap the burritos. Let cool to room temperature.

7. Wrap the burritos individually in plastic wrap for storing. Refrigerate for up to 3 days.

8. Divide the yogurt among 8 (2-ounce) cups with lids and the salsa among eight additional bowls with lids. Refrigerate with the burritos for up to 5 days.

Reheat:

If thawed, reheat burritos in the microwave for about 1 minute; if frozen, heat in the microwave for 1½ to 2 minutes, or until warm. Serve each with two tablespoons of salsa and two tablespoons of Greek yogurt on the side.

Freeze:

Transfer the wrapped burritos to a gallon-size resealable freezer bag and squeeze the air out before sealing. Freeze for up to 1 month — Thaw in the refrigerator overnight, or heat from frozen as directed.

Per serving (1 burrito with two tablespoons yogurt and two tablespoons salsa): Calories: 245; Fat: 9g; Protein: 23g; Total carbs: 23g; Net carbs: 15g; Fiber: 8g; Sugar: 5g; Sodium: 719mg

11. Fruity Quinoa Breakfast Bowl

Gluten-Free

Prep: 10 minutes | Cook: 9 minutes | Serves 3

Ingredients

- ✓ 1 cup pecans
- ✓ 2 tablespoons pure maple syrup
- ✓ 2 cups cooked red quinoa, cooled
- ✓ 1 cup diced fresh strawberries
- ✓ 1 cup fresh blueberries
- ✓ 1 (15-ounce) can mandarin oranges, drained
- ✓ ¼ cup raw honey
- ✓ 2 tablespoons freshly squeezed lime juice
- ✓ ½ teaspoon salt
- ✓ Dash ground cinnamon

Directions

1. Preheat the oven to 400°F. Line a small sheet pan with aluminum foil or a silicone mat. Set aside.

2. In a small bowl, stir together the pecans and maple syrup. Scrape the mixture onto the prepared sheet pan and spread it into a single layer. Bake for 7 to 9 minutes, flipping the nuts halfway through the baking time. Remove from the oven and let cool. (The pecans will harden as they cool.)

3. In a large bowl, stir together the quinoa, strawberries, blueberries, and oranges. Set aside.

4. In a small bowl, whisk the honey, lime juice, salt, and cinnamon. Add the dressing to the salad and mix to coat.

5. Divide the salad among three single-serving 24-ounce meal prep containers. Refrigerate for up to 3 days.

6. Break up the glazed pecans and divide them among three sandwich-size resealable bags—store at room temperature for up to 1 month.

7. When serving, top the quinoa and fruit with a sprinkle of glazed pecans.

Per serving (⅓ salad recipe with ⅓ cup pecans): Calories: 621; Fat: 29g; Protein: 11g; Total carbs: 89g; Net carbs: 78g; Fiber: 11g; Sugar: 52g; Sodium: 407mg

12. Chocolate Peanut Butter Smoothie

Dairy-Free, Gluten-Free, No Cook

Prep: 5 minutes | Serves 1

Ingredients

- ✓ ½ frozen banana
- ✓ ½ cup pasteurized egg whites
- ✓ 1 tablespoon natural peanut butter
- ✓ 1 cup unsweetened almond milk
- ✓ 1 scoop chocolate protein powder (whey or vegan)
- ✓ 1 cup of ice cubes

Directions

1. In a sandwich-size freezer bag, combine the banana, egg whites, and peanut butter. Freeze for up to 1 month.

2. In a high-powered blender, combine the freezer bag contents, milk, and protein powder. Blend on high speed for about 30 seconds.

3. Add the ice and blend for 30 seconds more, until smooth.

Per serving (1 shake): Calories: 304; Fat: 15g; Protein: 21g; Total carbs: 21g; Net carbs: 16g; Fiber: 5g; Sugar: 9g; Sodium:459mg

13. Spinach Breakfast Quesadilla

Nut-free

Prep: 5 minutes | cook: 10 minutes | serves 1

Ingredients

- ✓ Non-stick cooking spray
- ✓ ½ cup fresh spinach, chopped
- ✓ ⅓ cup egg whites or two large eggs
- ✓ Dash salt
- ✓ Dash freshly ground black pepper
- ✓ 1 flour tortilla
- ✓ 1-ounce shredded cheddar cheese
- ✓ 2 tablespoons salsa

Directions

1. Coat a medium-sized non-stick skillet with cooking spray and put it over medium heat.

2. Add the spinach and sauté for about 3 minutes, until wilted.

3. Pour the egg whites over the spinach and season with salt and pepper. Cook for 3 to 4 minutes, until the egg whites set. Fold the omelet in half. Carefully flip it and cook for 1 to 2 minutes more. Remove from the skillet and set aside on a plate.

4. Return the skillet to the heat and add the tortilla. Sprinkle it with the cheddar cheese. Cook for almost 1 to 2 minutes, until the cheese, melts, and transfer the tortilla to a plate.

5. Place the omelet on top of the cheese. Fold the tortilla in half and serve with the salsa.

6. For storage, wrap the quesadilla in plastic wrap. Put the salsa in a 2-ounce cup with a lid. Refrigerate for up to 3 days.

Reheat:

Unwrap the quesadilla before heating in the microwave for 30 to 40 seconds, or until heated thoroughly.

Per serving (1 quesadilla): calories: 221; fat: 10g; Protein: 18g; Total carbs: 14g; net carbs: 12g; fiber: 2g; Sugar: 2g; sodium: 427mg

14. Quick Apple Cinnamon Oatmeal

Dairy-free, gluten-free

Prep: 5 minutes | cook: 5 minutes | serves 3

Ingredients

cups water

1½ cups old-fashioned rolled oats

1 apple, diced (skin on)

1 tablespoon honey or sweetener of choice

2 tablespoons natural or powdered almond butter

One teaspoon ground cinnamon

Directions

1. In a medium saucepan over high heat, bring 3 cups water to a boil. Add the oats and apple. Cook for about 5 minutes, until the moisture is gone, frequently stirring to avoid sticking. Now, remove the pot from the stove, stir it in the honey, almond butter, and cinnamon.

2. Divide the oatmeal among three single-serving 24-ounce meal prep containers. Refrigerate for up to 6 days.

Reheat:

Reheat the oats for 1 minute in the microwave.

Freeze:

Once cooled, freeze the prepared oatmeal in 3 quart-size resealable freezer bags for up to 1 month. Thaw it overnight in your refrigerator and reheat as directed.

Per serving (1 container): calories: 319; fat: 12g; Protein: 8g; Total carbs: 48g; net carbs: 41g; fiber: 7g; Sugar: 15g; Sodium: 75mg

15. Vegetable Egg Muffins

Gluten-free, nut-free

Prep: 10 minutes | cook: 30 minutes | makes 18 muffins

Ingredients

- ✓ Non-stick cooking spray
- ✓ 6 large eggs
- ✓ 1 (16-ounce) carton egg whites
- ✓ 1½ cups shredded russet potato
- ✓ 1¼ cups meatless crumbles (such as boca brand)
- ✓ 1 cup chopped bell pepper, any color
- ✓ ½ cup shredded pepper jack cheese
- ✓ ¼ teaspoon salt
- ✓ ¼ teaspoon freshly ground black pepper

Directions

1. Preheat the oven to 350°f. Coat two muffin tins with cooking spray and set aside.

2. In a large bowl, whisk the whole eggs and egg whites for 30 seconds until fluffy. Pour ¼ cup of the egg mixture into each of 18 muffin tin wells.

3. In a medium bowl, stir together the potato, crumbles, bell pepper, jack cheese, salt, and pepper. Distribute the potato filling evenly on top of the egg filling.

4. Bake for 30 minutes, or until the centers are firm and a toothpick inserted into the center of a muffin comes out clean. Remove and let cool.

5. Put three muffins into each of 6 quart-size resealable bags. Refrigerate for up to 5 days.

Reheat:

Warm the muffins in the microwave for 45 seconds.

Freeze:

Freeze the muffins flat in a gallon-size resealable freezer bag for up to 1 month. Thaw in the refrigerator overnight and then reheat it as directed.

Per serving (3 muffins): calories: 181; fat: 8g; Protein: 20g; total carbs: 7g; net carbs: 6g; fiber: 1g; Sugar: 2g; sodium: 359mg

3.2 Quick to Eat Lunch Recipes

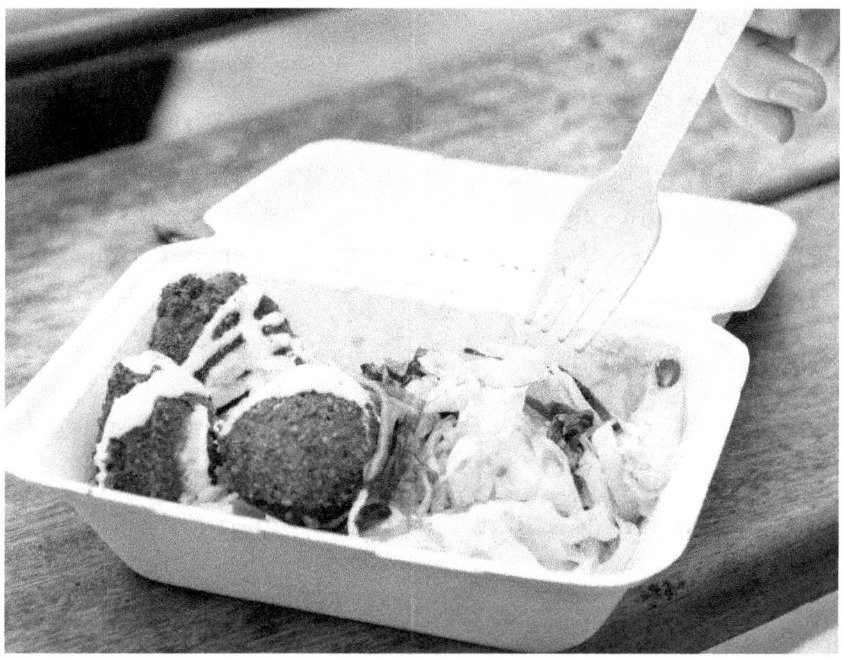

1. Caponata Pasta

prep: 2 mins | cook: 18 minutes | 4 serves

Nutrition per serving: Kcal 542 fat 14 g saturated 2 g carbs 85 g sugars 21 g Fiber 9 g Protein 14 g salt 0.5 g

Ingredients

- ✓ 4 tablespoons of olive oil
- ✓ 1 large onion (finely chopped)
- ✓ Four garlic cloves, finely sliced.
- ✓ 250 g of Mediterranean vegetation (peppers and aubergines, if possible) from the jar,
- ✓ Pot or deli counter
- ✓ Drained if in oil (you should use this oil instead of olive oil) and roughly chopped.
- ✓ 400 g can be chopped with tomatoes
- ✓ 1 tbsp of small capers

✓ 2 tablespoons raisins
✓ 350 g rigatoni, penne or other short pasta shapes
✓ Bunch of basil leaves.
✓ Parmesan (or vegetarian alternative), shaved, to eat.

Directions

1. Steam the oil in a large pan and cook the onion for 8-10 minutes before it begins to caramelize (or for longer if you have time – the sweeter, the better). Remove the garlic for the last 2 minutes of cooking time.

2. Tip in mixed fruits, onions, capers, and raisins. Season well and simmer, uncovered, for 10 minutes or until the sauce are rich.

3. Boil the kettle, meanwhile. Pour the kettleful of water in a large pan with a little salt and bring to a boil. Attach the pasta and cook until tender with a bit of crunch, then drain and save some of the water for the pasta. Tip the pasta in the sauce and apply a splash of water to the pasta if it needs to be loosened. Scatter with basil leaves and parmesan, if you like, and serve straight out of the pan.

2. Black Bean Burgers with Cilantro Greek Yogurt Spread

Nut-free

Prep: 25 minutes, plus 30 minutes to chill | cook: 10 minutes | makes six patties

Ingredients

✓ 1 recipe cilantro Greek yogurt spread, chilled
✓ 2 slices whole-wheat bread, toasted
✓ 2 tablespoons olive oil, divided
✓ One onion, chopped
✓ 2 garlic cloves, minced
✓ 2 tablespoons minced, seeded, and ribbed jalapeño pepper
✓ 1 teaspoon ground cumin

- ✓ 1 (15-ounce) can reduced-sodium black beans, drained and rinsed
- ✓ 1¼ cups cooked brown rice
- ✓ 1 teaspoon freshly squeezed lime juice
- ✓ ½ teaspoon salt
- ✓ ½ teaspoon freshly ground black pepper
- ✓ ¼ cup chopped fresh cilantro
- ✓ 1 head bibb lettuce
- ✓ 1 cucumber, sliced
- ✓ 1 tomato, sliced

Directions

1. Evenly divide the cilantro yogurt spread among 6 (2-ounce) cups with lids and set aside.

2. In a food processor, pulse the toasted bread to form crumbs. Transfer it to a small bowl and set aside.

3. In a large skillet over medium temperature, heat one tablespoon of olive oil. Add the onion, garlic, jalapeño, and cumin. Sauté for 2 minutes, stirring. Transfer the vegetables to the food processor.

4. Add the black beans, brown rice, lime juice, salt, and pepper to the processor. Pulse until the beans are rightly chopped but not puréed. Scrape the mixture into a large bowl and add half of the breadcrumbs and all of the cilantro. Stir until combined. Divide the dough into six portions, each about the size of a small baseball, and flatten them into patties. Put the patties over a baking sheet, cover them with plastic wrap, and refrigerate for 30 minutes, until firm.

5. Wipe out the skillet, put it over medium-high heat, and heat the remaining one tablespoon of olive oil. Add the patties and fry for almost 4 to 5 minutes per side, until firm. Transfer to paper towels to drain.

6. Wrap each patty in bibb lettuce and top with the cucumber and tomato. Put each burger into a single-serving 24-ounce meal prep container. Add one cilantro yogurt spread cup to each box. Refrigerate for up to 5 days.

Reheat:

Remove the patty from the container and unwrap it from the lettuce and vegetables. Heat the patty for 30 to 45 seconds in the microwave. Rewrap in the salad and top with the plants.

Freeze:

Freeze the uncooked patties in a single layer in a gallon- or quart-size freezer bag for up to 1 month. Defrost it in the refrigerator overnight afterward, cook it as directed.

Per serving (1 burger with vegetables and yogurt sauce): calories: 197; fat: 6g; Protein: 10g; total carbs: 31g; net carbs: 22g; fiber: 7g; Sugar: 4g; sodium: 329mg

3. Peanut Zoodle Salad

Dairy-free, no-cook

Prep: 15 minutes | serves 2

Ingredients

For the peanut sauce

- ✓ 2 tablespoons powdered peanut butter or natural peanut butter
- ✓ 2 tablespoons warm water
- ✓ 1½ tablespoons soy sauce
- ✓ 1 tablespoon honey
- ✓ 1 teaspoon sesame oil
- ✓ ½ teaspoon minced peeled fresh ginger

For the salad

- ✓ 10½ ounces zucchini spirals
- ✓ ½ cup shelled edamame

✓ ¼ large red bell pepper, sliced

✓ ¼ cup shredded carrot

✓ 2 tablespoons chopped scallion

✓ 2 tablespoons chopped fresh cilantro

Directions

To Make the Peanut Sauce:

In a small container, whisk the peanut butter, warm water, soy sauce, honey, sesame oil, and ginger until smooth. Set aside.

To Make the Salad:

In a large bowl, combine the zucchini, edamame, red bell pepper, carrot, and scallion.

Pour the peanut sauce over the zoodle mix and add the cilantro. Gently toss to mix. Evenly divide the salad between 2 (16-ounce) mason jars with lids. Seal the jars. Refrigerate for up to 4 days.

Per serving (1 jar): calories: 220; fat: 10g; Protein: 12g; total carbs: 24g; net carbs: 19g; fiber: 5g; Sugar: 15g; Sodium: 709mg

4. Kale and Sweet Potato Salad

Dairy-free option

Prep: 15 minutes | cook: 20 minutes | serves 2

Ingredients

For the Dressing

✓ 2 tablespoons apple cider vinegar
✓ 2 tablespoons olive oil
✓ 2 tablespoons freshly squeezed orange juice
✓ ¼ teaspoon salt
✓ ¼ teaspoon freshly ground black pepper, add more as needed

For the Salad

- ✓ Non-stick cooking spray
- ✓ One sweet potato, diced
- ✓ 2 tablespoons olive oil
- ✓ ½ teaspoon salt
- ✓ ¼ teaspoon freshly ground black pepper
- ✓ 3 cups finely chopped kale leaves
- ✓ ½ cup (dried) Israeli (also called pearl) couscous, cooked according to the package Directions.
- ✓ ⅓ cup dried low-sugar cranberries
- ✓ ⅓ cup toasted slivered almonds
- ✓ 2 ounces feta cheese, crumbled (optional)

Directions

1. Whisk the vinegar, olive oil, orange juice, salt, and pepper to make the dressing in a small bowl until combined. Set aside.

2. To make the salad, pre-heat the oven to 425°f. Lightly coat the baking sheet using some cooking spray.

3. On the baking sheet, toss the sweet potato, olive oil, salt, and pepper — Bake for 20 minutes, or until browned. Let cool on the baking sheet.

4. In a large bowl, combine the kale, couscous, cranberries, almonds, feta cheese, sweet potato, and dressing. Divide the salad between 2 single-serving 24-ounce meal prep containers. Refrigerate for up to 4 days.

Per serving (1 container): calories: 592; fat: 42g; Protein: 13g; total carbs: 46g; net carbs: 39g; fiber: 7g; Sugar: 8g; sodium: 1296mg

5. Vegetarian Taco Soup

Gluten-free

Prep: 15 minutes Cook: 3 hours serves 3 minutes

Ingredients

- ✓ 21/2 cups of water
- ✓ 1 (1-ounce) package taco seasoning
- ✓ 1 (1-ounce) pack of ranch dressing or two tablespoons of clean ranch seasoning
- ✓ No-salt-added diced tomatoes (15-ounce) cans with juice
- ✓ 1 (15.5-ounce) can be reduced-sodium black beans, drained and rinsed
- ✓ 1 (16-ounce) can be reduced-sodium pinto beans, drained and rinsed
- ✓ 1 cup of frozen white kernel corn
- ✓ 3/4 cup cheddar shredded cheddar cheese, divided
- ✓ 3/4 cup regular, non-fat Greek yogurt, divided
- ✓ Avocado strips, for serving (optional)

Directions

1. Combine water, taco seasoning, ranch dressing, tomatoes, black beans, pinto beans, and corn in a large pot over medium-high heat. Mix well, man. Bring your soup to a boil. Reduce heat to keep simmering, cover the pan, and cook for 3 hours. Taking the soup off the flame and let it cool down.

2. Place 1 cup of soup in each of 3 single-serve 24-ounce meal prep containers or 8-ounce mason jars with lids. Place 1/4 cup of cheddar cheese in each of 3 small boxes or sandwich resealable bags and 1/4 cup of yogurt in each of 3 small containers. Refrigerate cheese and yogurt with a meal of prep containers for up to 1 week.

3. When serving, add the avocado (if used).

4. Freeze any remaining soup in a resealable freezer bag, flat, for up to 2 months.

Reheat:

Heat the soup in the microwave in increments of 30 seconds, stirring until the desired temperature is reached.

Freeze:

To reheat, cook the soup in the refrigerator for at least 4 hours before reheating as directed.

Per serving (1 cup of 1/4 cup of cheese and 1/4 cup of yogurt): calories: 131; fat: 3 g; Protein: 8 g; total carbs: 15 g; Net carbs: 11 g; fiber: 4 g; sugar: 8 g; sodium: 491 mg

6. Margherita pizza pita

Nut-free

Prep: 5 minutes Cook: 10 minutes make six pizzas

Ingredients

- ✓ 6 pita bread
- ✓ No-salt-added tomato sauce will add 1 (8-ounce)
- ✓ Add 3 small tomatoes, thinly sliced.
- ✓ 1 cup of fresh basil leaves
- ✓ Eight ounces fresh mozzarella, sliced.
- ✓ 6 tablespoons of balsamic vinaigrette.

Directions

1. Preheat the oven to 350 degrees f. Fill a baking sheet of aluminum foil.

2. Put the pitas on the prepared baking sheet. Cover each with about two tablespoons of tomato sauce, three slices of tomato, two tablespoons of fresh basil leaves and 1/4 cup of mozzarella cheese.

3. Bake for 5 to 7 minutes, or until cheese is bubbled and melted. Let's just cool.

4. When it's cold, wrap every pizza in plastic wrap and a sheet of foil. Put two pizzas in each of three 24-ounce single-serve meal prep containers. Place two teaspoons of balsamic vinaigrette in each of 3 (2-ounce) cups with lids. Add one dressing container to every food prep bowl. Refrigerate the pizza and sauce for up to five days.

Reheat:

If you have access to an air fryer or toaster oven, you can hold the pita crisps. Warm at 390 ° f for about 2 minutes, until the cheese is lightly golden and bubbly. Cook for 1 minute more if necessary. If not, the microwave is just going to do fine. Reheat in intervals of 30 seconds until the target temperature is reached. Top with the balsamic dressing after the refrigeration.

Per serving (2 pizzas and 2 tablespoons of dressing): calories: 700; fat: 30 g; protein: 32 g; total carbs: 77 g; net carbs: 70 g; fiber: 7 g; sugar: 9 g; sodium: 1236 mg

7. Thai Noodle Bowls

Dairy-free

Prep: 20 minutes Cook: 15 minutes serve 2

Ingredients

In the Dressing

- ✓ 1/4 cup soy sauce
- ✓ 2 tablespoons of honey.
- ✓ 2 tablespoons of sesame oil
- ✓ Attach two cloves of garlic, minced
- ✓ Add 1/2 teaspoon filled with red pepper flakes.

For the Bowls

- ✓ 3 ounce of brown rice noodles
- ✓ 2 cups of bagged coleslaw mixture
- ✓ One scallion, sliced
- ✓ 1/2 red bell pepper, julienned
- ✓ 1/4 of a batch of fresh cilantro, chopped
- ✓ Add 1/2 tablespoon of jalapeno pepper.
- ✓ Add 1/4 cup crushed toasted peanuts.

Directions

1. To make the dressing, whisk the soy sauce, honey, sesame oil, garlic, and red pepper flakes in a small bowl until blended. Place it aside.

2. Cook the brown rice noodles following the package Directions to make the bowls. Drain, rinse with cold water, and drain while making the salad.

3. In a large bowl, add the coleslaw mixture, the scallion, the red bell pepper, the cilantro, the fried noodles, the jalapeño, and the peanuts. Well, toss to mix.

4. Divide the salad equally between two 24-ounce single-serve meal prep containers. Divide the dressing into 2 (2-ounce) cups with the lids. Inside the salad containers, place the dressing cups. Refrigerate the food for up to 4 days.

Per serving (1 container): calories: 416; fat: 23 g; protein: 9 g; total carbs: 50 g; net carbs: 44 g; fiber: 6 g; sugar: 24 g; sodium: 2007 mg;

8. Tomato Basil One-Pot Pasta

Gluten-free, dairy-free, nut-free

Prep: 10 minutes Cook: 30 minutes serves 4 minutes

Ingredients

- ✓ 1 (8-ounce) chickpea penne pasta kit
- ✓ 41/4 cups low-sodium vegetable broth
- ✓ No-salt-added diced tomatoes with juice 1 (15-ounce)
- ✓ 1/2 onion, chopped
- ✓ Add four cloves of garlic, thinly sliced.
- ✓ 2 tablespoons of olive oil
- ✓ 2 teaspoons of dried oregano
- ✓ 10 fresh basil leaves, roughly chopped.
- ✓ Salt
- ✓ Freshly ground black pepper.

Directions

1. In a big bowl, mix the pasta, vegetable broth, tomatoes, onion, garlic, olive oil, and oregano. Cover the pot and carry it to a boil. Reduce heat to keep simmering and cook for 20 minutes, stirring every few minutes.

2. Stir in basil, season with salt and pepper. Let's just cool.

3. Divide the pasta evenly into four 24-ounce single-serve meal prep containers. Refrigerate for up to five days. This meal doesn't freeze very well.

Reheat:

Reheat the pasta in the microwave for about 45 seconds or until it reaches the target temperature.

Per serving (1 container): calories: 320; fat: 11 g; protein: 18 g; total carbs: 43 g; net carbs: 32 g; fiber: 11 g; sugar: 11 g; sodium: 208 mg

9. Soup Butternut Squash

Gluten privileges

Prep: 15 minutes Cook: 8 hours serve 3 minutes

Ingredients

- ✓ 1 butternut squash, halved, seeds and pulp removed, peeled, and diced
- ✓ 2 celery stalks, cut into small dice
- ✓ 1 white onion, diced
- ✓ 1 granny smith apple, cored and diced
- ✓ 2 garlic cloves, minced
- ✓ 2 cups of low-sodium vegetable broth
- ✓ 1/2 teaspoon of salt, more as required
- ✓ 1/4 teaspoon of black pepper freshly ground, plus more as needed.
- ✓ 1/4 teaspoon ground cinnamon.
- ✓ 1/4 teaspoon ground nutmeg.
- ✓ 1/8 teaspoon, plus more as needed cayenne pepper

- ✓ 1 bay leaf
- ✓ One fresh, sage leaf.
- ✓ 1/2 cup canned lite milk for cocoa
- ✓ 1/2 cup plain nonfat Greek yogurt.

Directions

1. Combine squash, cellar, onion, apple, garlic, vegetable squash, salt, black pepper, cinnamon, and cayenne with a slow cooker. Delete to blend. Top with the sage and the lake leaf.

2. Cover and cook on low heat for 6 to 8 hours and on high heat for 3 to 4 hours till the squash is tender and easy to mash with a fork.

3. Remove the bay leaf and sage and discard it. Mix the coconut milk and yogurt.

4. Mix the soup in the slow cooker with an immersion blender. Instead, work in tons, move the soup to a regular blender, and purée to a smooth finish. Let cool. Let cool.

5. Divide the soup evenly into three single-serving 24-ounce preparation containers. Suitable for up to 1 week.

Reheat:

Reheat the soup for 1 minute or until the temperature you want is reached.

Freeze:

This soup is ideal for busy nights when you need a fast meal. Freeze the soup for up to 2 months in a resealable freezer bag, flat. Thaw overnight in the refrigerator and reheat as directed.

Per serving (1 container): 245 calories, 3 g fat, 9 g protein, total carbon: 52 g, 42 g net carbs, 10 g fiber, 17 g sugar, 384 mg sodium.

10. Salad Tuscan Chickpea

No cook, no gluten-free, nut-free

Prep: 20 min serves 4

Ingredients

For the Dressing

- ✓ 1/4 cup of olive oil.
- ✓ 2 tablespoons non-fat Greek yogurt
- ✓ One tablespoon of freshly squeezed citrus fruit juice
- ✓ One tablespoon of vinegar red wine
- ✓ 1 small clove of garlic
- ✓ 1/4 teaspoon ground cumin.
- ✓ Salt
- ✓ Black pepper freshly ground.

For the Salad

- ✓ 2(15-ounce) cans of chickpeas of reduced sodium, drained and rinsed
- ✓ 1 cup of canned artichoke heart
- ✓ 3/4 cup of grape-half tomatoes.
- ✓ 3 scallions, cut.
- ✓ 2/3 cup yellow bell pepper chopped
- ✓ Tomatoes with 1/3 cup of sun-dried, diced
- ✓ 1/3 cup of cheese feta, crumbled.
- ✓ 1/4 of a cup of fresh Italian parsley
- ✓ 1 skin red leaf lettuce, washed, chopped and dried thoroughly

Directions

1. In a small bowl, mix olive oil, cream, lemon juice, vinegar, garlic, and cumin to make the dressing. Taste salt and pepper and season. Whisk to blend again. Set aside. Set aside.

2. Toss the chickpeas, artichoke heart, onions, scallions, bell pepper, sun-dried onions, feta cheese, and parsley in a big bowl to make the salad.

3. Split the red leaf lettuce equally into four 24-ounce single-serve ready meal containers. Top each with a fourth of the mixture of chickpeas. Spread the dressing uniformly between four (2-ounce) cups and placed them in the salad containers. Hot for up to 4 days.

Serving (1 bowl): 299 calories; 17 g fat; 11 g protein; 31 g total carbs; 26 g net carbon; 5 g fiber; 11 g sugar; 436 mg sodium;

11. Roasted Brussels Sprouts Salad

Prep: 20 min Cook: 50 min serve 4

Ingredients

For the Dressing

- ✓ ½ cup of sliced fresh strawberries.
- ✓ 2 tablespoons of olive oil.
- ✓ 2 tablespoons apple cider vinegar
- ✓ Two tablespoons of raw honey, or pure maple syrup
- ✓ 1/2 teaspoon salt.
- ✓ 1/4 of teaspoon freshly ground black pepper

For the Glazed Pecans

- ✓ Half cup of pecan or walnut.
- ✓ 3 tablespoons of pure maple syrup.

For the salad

- ✓ 1-pound sprouts in Brussels, trimmed
- ✓ One tablespoon of olive oil.

✓ One head romaine lettuce washed and chopped
✓ 2 cups baby kale
✓ 1 cup of diced cucumber
✓ 1/2 cup of violet raisin, half-cooked.
✓ 1/4 cup of fresh blueberries.
✓ ¼ cup purple grapes or low-sugar dried cranberries
✓ 1/4 cup of feta, crumbled cheese.
✓ 1/4 cup red onion diced
✓ 1/3 cup of pepitas if needed toasted.

Directions

To make the Dressing

Combine the strawberries, olive oil, vinegar, sugar, salt, and pepper in a strong blender. Puree until smooth. Puree divide the dressing equally into 4 (2-ounce) cups and set aside.

To make the pecans glazed

1. Preheat the microwave oven to a temperature of 350 ° f. Line a small sheet of paper and set aside.

2. Cut the pecans and maple syrup together in a small bowl until they are powdered. Scrap the pecan mixture on the prepared sheet pot and stretch it into one layer.

3. Bake until glazed for 5 to 7 minutes. Remove and allow to harden to cool. Divide the glazed pecans into four snack bags. Set aside.

For the salad

1. Raise the temperature of the oven to 425 ° f.

2. Combine brussels sprouts and olive oil on a baking sheet or sheet pan with a coat. Rub for 35 to 40 minutes until golden brown and slightly crispy at the tops of the sprouts. Let cool.

3. Toss lettuce and kale together in a big bowl. Divide the greens into four 24-ounce single-serving meal preparation containers.

4. Combine sprouts, cucumber, raisins, blueberries, raisins, feta cheese, red onion, and pepitas in a large bowl. Flip to mix. Divide the mixture from Brussels equally between the four meal prep containers over the vegetables. In each salad bowl, add one dressing cup and one bag of pecans.

5. Add the nuts and the dressing before food to the salad. Cool the containers up to 4 days.

Per serving: calories: 510; fat: 23 g; protein: 10 g; total carbs: 77 g; net carbs: 67 g; fiber: 10 g; sugar: 50 g; sodium: 395 mg.

12. Sweet Potatoes Loaded Veggie

Gluten-free

Prep: 10 min Cook: 40 min serves 3

Ingredients

- ✓ 3 Large sweet potatoes
- ✓ 3/4 cup canned red-sodium black beans, drained and rinsed
- ✓ 3/4 cup enchilada sauce or clean enchilada sauce
- ✓ 1/2 tablespoon of chili powder
- ✓ 1/2 teaspoon of salt
- ✓ 1/2 teaspoon of ground cumin
- ✓ 11/2 cups of cottage cheese
- ✓ 1 avocado, peel on, pitted, and quartered

Directions

1. Preheat the oven at 400 ° f temperature.

2. Place the sweet potatoes over a baking sheet and cook for 40 minutes or until they are easily pierced with a fork. Put it aside and let it cool.

3. Split the sweet potatoes lengthwise without going all the way into it. Slowly scoop out of the center, leaving a border of sweet potato around the edges.

4. In a medium cup, mix sweet potatoes, black beans, enchilada sauce, chili powder, salt, and cumin. Stir well and mix well. Fill each sweet potato with one-third of the filling of the black bean.

5. Put one sweet potato in each of 3 24-ounce single-serve meal prep containers. Add 1/2 cup of cottage cheese in each of 3 small airtight containers. Wrap the avocado quarters individually in plastic wrap and insert one quarter in each of the three resealable sandwich bags. Add one box of cottage cheese and one packet of avocado to each container of sweet potatoes. Put the remaining quarter of the avocado in a delightful potato bowl or refrigerator. Refrigerate for up to five days.

Reheat:

Heat the stuffed sweet potatoes in a microwave for 2 minutes or in a 350 ° f oven for 10 minutes. Add the cottage cheese and the avocado just before serving.

Per serving (1 stuffed sweet potato, 1/2 cup cottage cheese, and one-quarter avocado): calories: 326; fat: 10 g; Protein: 15 g; total carbs: 48 g; Net carbs: 35 g; fiber: 13 g; sugar: 8 g; sodium: 554 mg

13. Tofu Wraps Lettuce

Dairy-free, vegan

Prep: 15 minutes Cook: 15 minutes serves 4 minutes

Ingredients

- ✓ 3 Ounces of Tofu Drained and Pressed
- ✓ 1/4 Teaspoon of Salt.
- ✓ 1/4 Teaspoon of Grounded Black Pepper.
- ✓ 1 Cup of Roughly Chopped Onion
- ✓ 4 Garlic Cloves, Minced.
- ✓ 1 (1-Inch) Piece of Fresh Ginger, Minced, And Peeled.
- ✓ 3/4 Cup of Water to The Chestnuts, Drained and Roughly Chopped.
- ✓ 3 Tablespoons of Hoisin Sauce

- ✓ One Tablespoon of Soy Sauce
- ✓ 1/2 Cup of Shredded Carrot
- ✓ 4 Tablespoons of Roughly Chopped Peanuts
- ✓ Two Tablespoons of Toasted Sesame Seeds.
- ✓ Four Tablespoons of Chopped Scallion
- ✓ 12 Bibb Lettuce Leaves

Directions

1. Spray a large skillet using a cooking spray and position over medium-high heat. Connect the tofu to that. Using a spatula or a large spoon, cut it into smaller pieces. Season to taste with pepper and salt and cook for 5 minutes. Transfer to the plate set aside.

2. Return to normal-high heat and add the onion, garlic, and ginger. Just sauté for 3 to 4 minutes

3. Stir in the tofu, the water chestnuts, the hoisin sauce, and the soy sauce. Cook to warm for about 3 minutes, then set aside to cool.

4. Divide the tofu mixture evenly between 4 24-ounce single-serve meal prep containers. In each dish, put two tablespoons of carrot, one tablespoon of peanuts, two teaspoons of sesame seeds, and one tablespoon of scallion.

5. Place three lettuce leaves in 4 different resealable bags or on top of each salad. If you want to reheat the tofu mixture, store the tofu mixture separately. Place the lettuce cups on a plate and top with the tofu mixture when ready to eat.

Reheat:

This dish is excellent served cold, but you can also heat the tofu mixture (without the toppings) in the microwave for 30 to 45 seconds.

Freeze:

Freeze the mixture of tofu in a quart-sized resealable freezer bag, flat, for up to 1 month. Defrost it in the refrigerator overnight afterward, reheat it as instructed, adding additional Ingredients to serve.

Calories: 173; fat: 8 g; protein: 7 g; total carbs: 21 g; net carbs: 18 g; fiber: 3 g; sugar: 7 g; sodium: 587 mg

14. Rainbow Wraps

Dairy-free, cook, nut-free, vegan

Prep: 10 min serves 3

Ingredients

- ✓ 3 low-carb wraps, with any taste.
- ✓ Six tablespoons of hummus
- ✓ 3 cups of fresh spinach leaves
- ✓ 1 1/2 cups of shredded carrot
- ✓ Six tablespoons of red onion.
- ✓ Six tablespoons of sunflower seeds.
- ✓ 1 1/2 cups of sliced red bell pepper
- ✓ 1 cup alfalfa sprouts or bean sprouts

Directions

1. Put the wraps on the surface of the job. Place two tablespoons of hummus on each cover. Top each wrap with 1 cup of spinach, 1/2 cup of carrot, two tablespoons of red onion, two tablespoons of sunflower seed, 1/2 cup of red bell pepper, and 1/3 cup of alfalfa sprouts.

2. Stretch the sides of the wraps, then roll up like a burrito.

3. Wrap each burrito individually in plastic wrap and place 1 in each of 3 24-ounce single-serve meal prep containers. Refrigerate for up to five days.

Per serving (1 wrap): calories: 224; fat: 8 g; protein: 14 g; total carbs: 35 g; net carbs: 20 g; fiber: 15 g; sugar: 7 g; sodium: 494 mg

15. Potato Sweet and Black Bean Enchiladas

Nut-free

Prep: 25 minutes Cook: 1 hour serves 4 minutes

Ingredients

- ✓ Non-stick cooking spray
- ✓ One tablespoon of olive oil
- ✓ One yellow onion, diced
- ✓ 1 teaspoon of chili powder.
- ✓ One teaspoon of ground cumin.
- ✓ 1/2 teaspoon of salt.
- ✓ 2 Sweet potatoes, cut into 1-inch cubes.
- ✓ 1/4 cup of water
- ✓ 1 (15-ounce)-sodium black beans, drained and rinsed
- ✓ 8 corn tortillas
- ✓ 1 Clean enchilada sauce or storage-bought sauce
- ✓ 11/2 cups of shredded white cheddar cheese

Directions

1. Preheat the oven to 350 degrees f. Coat a 9-by-13-inch baking dish with a hot spray.

2. Heat the oil in a normal-sized pan over normal-high heat. Attach the onion and sauté for about four minutes, until softened.

3. In the chili powder, the cumin, and the oil. Cook for about 1 minute. Add some sweet potatoes and water. Cover the skillet and cook for 12 minutes.

4. Stir the black beans and cook for almost 5 to 6 minutes or until the sweet potatoes are tender.

5. While the sweet potatoes and black beans are cooked, cover the corn tortillas in a damp paper towel and heat in the microwave for 1 to 2 minutes or until they are slightly foldable.

6. Fill single tortilla with 1⁄2 cup of sweet potato filling and top with a spoonful of enchilada sauce. Roll up your tortillas. Don't worry about the side folding. It's all right if the Ingredients spill out.

7. Place the enchiladas in the prepared baking dish and top with the desired amount of enchilada sauce. Top with cheddar cheese and cook for 25 to 30 minutes, until the cheese is bubbly and lightly browned.

8. Remove from the oven and let it cool down.

9. Put two enchiladas in each of 3 24-ounce single-serve meal prep containers. Refrigerate for about five days.

Reheat:

Heat the enchiladas in the microwave for 1 minute.

Freeze:

They freeze well. Place the enchiladas in a resealable freezer bag and freeze, flat, for up to 1 month. Thaw overnight in the refrigerator and reheat as directed.

Per serving (2 enchiladas): calories: 394; fat: 17 g; Protein: 17 g; total carbs: 45 g; Net carbs: 36 g; fiber: 9 g; sugar: 5 g; sodium: 474 mg;

3.3 Ready to Cook and Warm Dinner Recipes

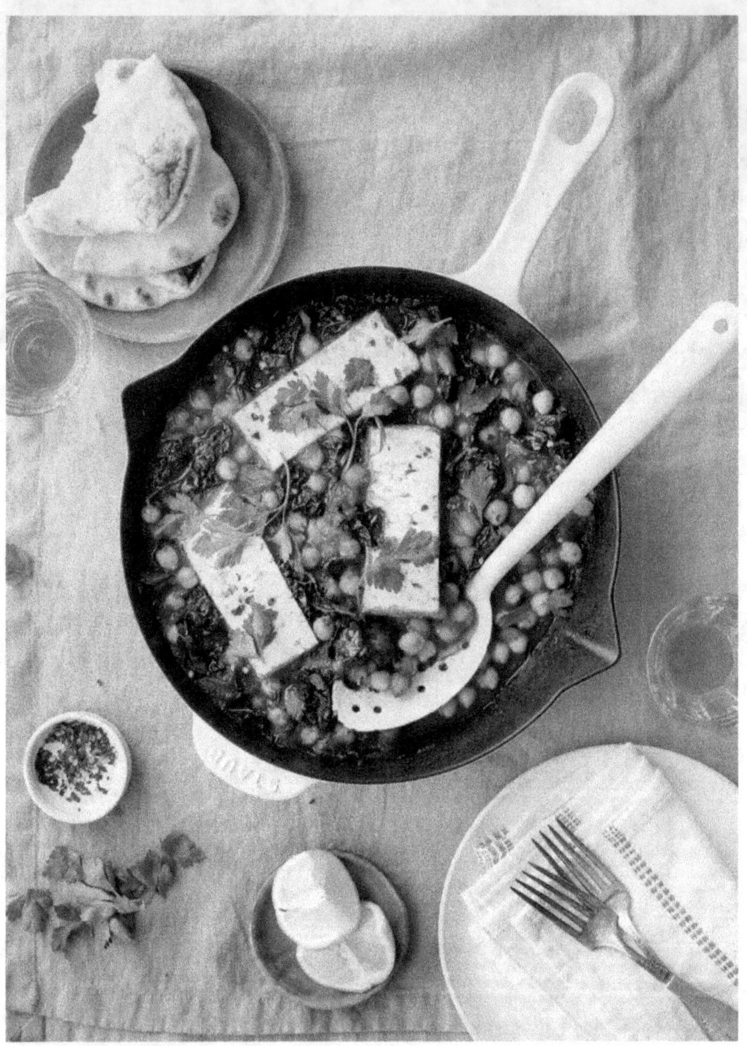

1. Three-Bean Cassoulet

Serving 2 prep 11/2 bowls

Calory: 304 mg Fat: 1.5 g fat Carbon dioxide: 58 g Protein: 21 g Fiber: 13 g Sugar: 16 g 819 mg of sodium.

Ingredients

- ✓ 1 garlic
- ✓ Fresh snap beans for 4 ounces.
- ✓ One zucchini
- ✓ 1/3 cup of white onion chopped
- ✓ Around 1 cup roman beans (also referred to as flat Italian beans)
- ✓ 3/4 cup of peas is black-eyed.
- ✓ One tomato sauce.
- ✓ 1 cup of broth of vegetables.
- ✓ One teaspoon dried parsley flake.
- ✓ 1/2 teaspoon dried basil.
- ✓ 1/2 teaspoon (or to taste) salt.

Directions

1. Preheat the oven to 350 ° f. Preheat.

2. Smash the garlic clove, peel, and chop. Wash and rinse the snap beans. Cut the ends and cut any brown spots off. Wash, peel, slice the zucchini.

3. Take a bowl of boiling water. Blanch the snap beans for 3 minutes in the boiling water until bright green.

4. In a non-grated 11/2 to 2 quarters casserole dish, combine the garlic, snap beans, turquoise, onion, Romano beans, black-eyed peas, tomato sauce, and chicken broth.

5. Cut dried pear, dried basil, and salt from the mixture.

6. Bake 2–21/2 hours until vegetables are tender and cassoulet thickened, whisking occasionally.

2. Vegetarian Cabbage Rolls

Yields 10 rolls Five rolls (2 serving rolls)

Calory: 186 Fat: 7 grams Carbohydrates: 23 g carbohydrates Protein: 9 g protein Fiber: 5 g Sugar: 15 g 493 mg of sodium

Ingredients

- ✓ 6 ounces firm tofu

- ✓ 2 teaspoons of olive oil
- ✓ Take one garlic diaper, chopped
- ✓ 1/2 red ointment, hacked
- ✓ 1 cup of tomatoes crushed
- ✓ Two and half black bell pepper.
- • 1/2 teaspoon ground cumin.
- ✓ 1/8 teaspoon (or to taste) paprika
- ✓ ten boiled cabbage leaves
- ✓ 6 ounces of sauce tomato.
- ✓ 2 ounces of water.
- ✓ 2 tablespoons of white vinegar.
- ✓ Two teaspoons of granular sugar

Directions

1. Preheat the oven to 350 ° f. Preheat. Sprinkle a large bakery with non-stick spray.

2. Drain into small pieces the tofu and dice. In a medium-sized skillet, heat the oil. Add onion and garlic. Salt until the onion is soft. Crumble the tofu into the bowl. Add the tomatoes and the green pepper and spatula to the tomatoes to break them up. Combine cumin and paprika in the forest.

3. Put a cod leaf flat on the counter. Disseminate two heaping tablespoons of middle fill (exact quantity required depends on cabbage leaf size). Roll up the bottom, tuck the sides and roll up to the top. Place the roll in the bakery plate with the seeded on the bottom.

4. Mix tomato sauce, water, white vinegar, and sugar in a small cup. Pour over the rolls of cod. Bake the cotton rolls in the oven for 40–45 minutes.

3. Tofu Sesame Baked

Serving 6 Through 4-oz. Calory: 93 Fat: 6 g Carbs: 3 g carbohydrates Food: 8 g protein Fiber: 1 g Sugar: 1 g 418 mg sodium

Ingredients

- ✓ 1/4 Cup (Low Sodium) Soy Sauce.
- ✓ Sesame Oil 2 Tablespoons.
- ✓ 3/4 Teaspoon Paste of Garlic.
- ✓ 1/2 Teaspoon Paste of Ginger
- ✓ 2 Blocks Firm Tofu Sticks, Well Pressed

Directions

1. Stir in soy, sesame oil, garlic, and ginger powder together and transfer to a wide, shallow bowl. Slice the tofu into 1/2-inch bands or triangles. Place the tofu in a plastic bag and add the marinade to the refrigerator. Marinate for 1 hour or overnight.

2. Preheat oven to 400 degrees f. Cover a pan with non-stick spray or olive oil, or foil rows. Place the tofu on the sheet.

3. Bake 20–25 minutes, turn over, then bake 10–15 minutes or until done.

4. Tofu marinating

5. A zipper top bag will help marinate cooked tofu dishes to make the tofu well coated with the marinade. Put the tofu in the bag, pour it in the marinade, seal, put on a fridge, and turn and shake lightly to coat every side of the tofu from time to time.

4. Tofu Fast Fried

Serving 3 By 3/4 of a cup Calory: 132 Fat: 10 grams Carbs: 8 g carbohydrates Protein: 9 g protein Fiber: 2 g Sugar: 15 g 208 mg of sodium

Ingredients

- ✓ 1 extra-strong tofu block, cubed
- ✓ 1/4 tablespoon soy sauce
- ✓ Two tablespoons of maize
- ✓ 2 Tablespoon nutritional yeast
- ✓ One teaspoon of powdered garlic

- ✓ 1/4 teaspoon oil
- ✓ Dash pepper
- ✓ 1/4 of the cup of frying oil

Directions

1. Marinate for at least 1 hour in soy sauce.

2. Combine meal, nutritional yeast, garlic powder, salt, and pepper in a small bowl.

3. Coat tofu well and flour mixture on both sides, fry in hot oil for about 4-5 minutes until slightly golden brown on both sides.

5. Lemon Basil Tofu

Serving 6 Per 3 or 4 oz slices. Tofu's Calories: 130 calories Fat: 7 grams Carbs: 11 g carbohydrates Food: 10 g protein Fiber: 6 g Sugar: 1.5 g 398 mg of sodium

Ingredients

- ✓ 3 Tablespoon of Citrus Juice
- ✓ One Tablespoon of Soy Sauce
- ✓ 2 Tablespoons Apple Cider Vinegar for Teaspoons
- ✓ Dijon Mustard for One Tablespoon
- ✓ 3/4 Teaspoon Sugar.
- ✓ 3 Tablespoon of Olive Oil.
- ✓ 2 Tablespoons Chopped Basil, Plus Additional Garnish
- ✓ Extra-Firm Tofu In 2 Blocks, Well Pressed

Directions

1. Whisk all Ingredients together, except tofu, and transfer to a bakery or casserole bowl.

2. Slice the tofu into 1/2-inch bands or triangles. Place the marinade with the tofu and cover it well. Allow to marinate for at least 1 hour or overnight, tofu is well marinated.

3. Preheat the oven to 350 ° f. Preheat. Switch over for 15 minutes, then bake for 10–12 minutes or until done. Add a few extra pieces of fresh chopped basil.

6. Simple Parmigiana Eggplant

Serves four 1/4 of the recipe Calories: 173; Fats: 9 carbohydrate: 11 g Protein: 11 g Fiber: 3 g Sugar: 6 g of sugar Sodium: 573 mg

Ingredients

- ✓ 1 medium eggplant
- ✓ 1/2 teaspoon of dried basil.
- ✓ 1/2 teaspoon of dried oregano.
- ✓ 1/8 teaspoon of garlic salt.
- ✓ 1 cup of spaghetti sauce
- ✓ Four slices of mozzarella cheese
- ✓ 1/4 cup grated parmesan cheese

Directions

1. Pre-heat the oven to 350 ° f. Spray an 8″ × 8″ non-stick cooking spray pans.

2. Wash the eggplant and then cut it into 1/4-inch-thick slices. Stir in the spaghetti sauce the dried basil, dried oregano, and garlic salt.

3. Place half the slices of the eggplant flat on the prepared baking pan. Place the spaghetti sauce over the top. Cover the eggplant with foil and cook for 20 minutes or until tender. Delete it from the oven. Uncover the slices of mozzarella and lay them on top.

4. Bake another 3–5 minutes until the cheese has melted. Sprinkle with parmesan cheese and serve well.

7. Tofu Palak, Indian

Serves 4 Per 1 cup of serving Calories: 55 Fats: 10 g Carbohydrate: 16 g Protein: 15 g of Fiber: 8 g Sugar: 2 g Sodium, 597 mg

Ingredients

- ✓ 3 garlic leaves, minced.
- ✓ One block of firm tofu, cut into small cubes.

✓ 2 teaspoons of olive oil
✓ Add two teaspoons of nutritional yeast.
✓ 1/2 tablespoon of onion powder
✓ 4 bunches of fresh spinach
✓ Three teaspoons of water
✓ One tablespoon of curry powder
✓ Two teaspoons of cumin.
✓ 1/2 teaspoon of salt.
✓ 1/2 cup plain soy yogurt

Directions

1. Steam the garlic and tofu in the olive oil over low heat, add the dietary yeast and the onion powder and stir to cover the tofu. Cook for 2-3 minutes until tofu is lightly browned.

2. Remove spinach, tea, curry, cumin, and salt and mix well to blend. When spinach begins to wilt, add soy yogurt and heat until spinach is thoroughly wilted and soft.

8. Tofu BBQ "Steaks" Sauce

Three serves Per 10 oz. Serve Calories: 240 cm Fats: 13 g Carbohydrate: 19 g Protein: 11 g Fiber: 1 g Sugar: 13 g Sodium: 885 mg

Ingredients

✓ 1/3 cup barbecue sauce
✓ 1/4 cup of water
✓ 2 teaspoons of balsamic vinegar
✓ 2 tablespoons of soy sauce
✓ Add 1–2 tablespoons of hot sauce (or to taste)
✓ Add two teaspoons of sugar.
✓ 2 blocks extra-firm tofu, well pressed
✓ 1/2 onion, chopped
✓ Two tablespoons of olive oil

Directions

1. In a small container, whisk together the barbecue sauce, water, vinegar, soy sauce, hot sauce, and sugar until well blended. Place it aside.

2. Break pressed tofu into 1/4-inch thick sheets.

3. In butter, sauté the onions and carefully add the tofu. Fry tofu on both sides until it is lightly golden brown, about two minutes on each side.

4. Reduce heat and apply a mixture of barbecue sauce, stirring to cover the tofu well. Cook over medium-low heat until sauce is absorbed and thickened for about 5–6 minutes.

5. Tofu versus seitan

6. Like other pan-fried or stir-fried tofu recipes, this recipe will also work well with seitan, but seitan needs a little longer to cook all the way through; otherwise, it will end up hard and chewy. Seitan is not typically more costly, but it can be more challenging to locate.

9. Manchego-Potato Tacos with Pickled Jalapenos

Serves 8 For one taco Calories: 207; Fats: 11 g Carbohydrate: 18 g

Protein: 7 g Fiber: 3 g Sugar: 1 g Sodium: 402 mg of

Ingredients

- ✓ 1 cup leftover mashed potatoes
- ✓ 8 soft corn tortillas
- ✓ 1/4 pound of Spanish mancheron cheese, cut into 16 small sticks.
- ✓ Pickled 16 slices of jalapeño pepper (available in Mexican parts and ethnic specialty stores)
- ✓ Four tablespoons of unsalted butter

Directions

1. Spoon 1 tablespoon of the mashed potato in the middle of each tortilla. Flatten the potatoes, leaving a margin of 1-inch. Lay 2 pieces of manchego and two pieces of jalapeño pickled on each tortilla, then fold it in a half-moon shape.

2. Melt half of the butter in a skillet over medium heat. Gently put four tacos in the pan and cook until well browned, around 3–4 minutes on each hand. Drain the paper towels. Repeat the remaining tacos. Snip the tacos in half before serving the salsa.

10. Ratatouille and Cannellini Beans

Serves six for 1 cup Calories: 167; Fats: 5 g Carbohydrate: 24 g Protein: 8 g of Fiber: 8 g

Sugar: 8 g of sugar Sodium 405 mg

Ingredients

- ✓ 2 tablespoons of olive oil
- ✓ One big onion, diced
- ✓ 2 medium zucchinis, diced
- ✓ 2 medium yellow squash, diced.
- ✓ One tiny eggplant, diced
- ✓ One bell pepper, diced
- ✓ 2 cups of cannellini beans, cooked
- ✓ One tablespoon flour
- ✓ 3 tomatoes, seeded, and cut into 6 bits.
- ✓ Two teaspoons of dried herbs of Provence (or a mixture of oregano, thyme, rosemary, marjoram, savory or lavender)
- ✓ Add one tablespoon of salt.
- ✓ Freshly ground black pepper.

Directions

1. Heat the olive oil in a heavy-bottomed Dutch oven until it is dry, but not smoky. Add the onion; cook until translucent, about five minutes. Within a large paper bag, add the zucchini, the yellow squash, the eggplant, and the bell pepper; the dust with the flour, the folding bag closed, and shake to coat. Add floured vegetables, onions, spices, salt, and pepper to the bowl.

2. Reduce heat to a boil, cover, and cook gently for 1 hour, until all vegetables are tender. Serve hot or damp at room temperature.

11. Eggplant Rollatini

Serving 8 Per 1 roller Calory: 339 fat: 13-gram Carbs: 34 g carbohydrates Protein: 22 grams Fiber: 6 g Sugar: 8 g 856 mg of sodium.

Ingredients

- ✓ 1 big eggplant, sliced in just 1/8-inch longitudes (as thick as a book cover)
- ✓ Flour to dredge
- ✓ Egg wash of 6 beaten eggs, mixed with 1/2 cup water
- ✓ 2 cups bread crumbs
- ✓ Oil for frying
- ✓ 1 pound of ricotta from
- ✓ 8 ounces of mozzarella ground cheese
- ✓ 1/2 cup of parmesan grated
- ✓ Salt and pepper.
- ✓ Fresh spinach, washed and cooked, 11/2 pounds.
- ✓ 4 tomato sauce cups

Directions

1. Bread and fry the eggplant: dip one piece of eggplant into the flour, cover it on both sides; shake off excess flour, wash it in the egg, shake it out, and coat it into bread chips to keep it tightly.

Place on a rack and repeat with remaining pieces. Heat oil to 350 ° f. Fry the breaded eggplant pieces for 1 minute per side and drip off any excess fat before stuck between layers of towels.

2. Filling and rolling: 350 ° f heat oven. In a mixing bowl, combine the three slices of cheese and lightly season with salt and pepper. At the wide end of the fried aubergines, place one teaspoon cooked spinach and a generous teaspoon of cheese mix. Roll away from yourself, jellyroll, and put the seam on the bottom of the bakery. Repeat with remaining aubergines and fillings and close the finished roulades in a bakery.

3. Bake until the cheeses are hot, and the edges start to lightly brown. Serve with basil leaves in a bowl of tomato sauce — one piece per portion of aperitif, 2 per the main course.

12. Grilled Marinated Mushrooms of Portobello

Serving per 1 champagne. Calories: 100 calories Fat: 7 grams Carbon dioxide: 7 protein: 3 g protein Fiber: 2 sugar: 5 gouda: 462 mg

Ingredient

- ✓ Four large mushrooms of portobello (4–6 inches in diameter) remove stem
- ✓ One taste of extra virgin olive oil.
- ✓ 1 cup of vinegar red wine
- ✓ 2 cucumbers with soy sauce.
- ✓ One Kochhar of sugar.
- ✓ 1/2 cup of chopped fresh cabbage.

Directions

1. Brush the mushrooms with clay, but don't wash them underwater. Whisk olive oil, vinegar, soy sauce, sugar, and cabbage together. Pour the marinade over the champagne in a shallow dish; marinate for 10 minutes, turning periodically.

2. Grill on each side for 2–3 minutes. Serve in full or in sliced form. Sauce with marinade remaining or save another batch of the marinade.

13. Chile's Black Bean and Butternut Squash

Serving 4Per 11⁄2 bowls Calory: 339Fat: 8g fat: Carbon dioxide: 55gProtein: 16g protein fiber: 16 g Sugar: 12 g

Ingredients

- ✓ One onion, chopped
- ✓ 3 cloves of garlic, chopped
- ✓ 2 tablespoons of oil.
- ✓ One medium squash of butternut, chopped into pieces
- ✓ 2 15-ounce tins of raw, drained, and rinsed beans.
- ✓ Tomatoes can be diced, untrained by one 28-ounce.
- ✓ 3⁄4 cup of vegetable bouillon.
- ✓ 1 tablespoon chili powder
- ✓ One tablespoon cumin.
- ✓ 1/4 teaspoon of cayenne pepper
- ✓ 1⁄2 teaspoon oil!
- ✓ Two tablespoons of fresh cilantro chopped.

Directions

1. Sprinkle onion and garlic in oil in a large stock until soft, around 4 minutes. Reduce heat and dd other Ingredients except for coriander.

2. Cover and cook for 25 minutes. Cover. Uncover and cook 5 minutes more. Just before serving, cover with fresh cilantro.

14. Tofu Fillet Beer-Battered

Serving 8through 6-oz. Service Calory: 289Fat: 16 g Carbs: 21 g carbohydrates Food: 12 g protein Fiber: 1 g fiber Sugar: 1.4 g.306 mg sodium.

Ingredients

- ✓ 2 teaspoons ground garlic.

- ✓ 2 powdered teaspoons onion
- ✓ Two teaspoons of peppers.
- ✓ 1 tablespoon of salt.
- ✓ 1/2 teaspoon black pepper.
- ✓ 3 extra-firm tofu blocks cut into chunks
- ✓ 1 12-ounce beer bottle
- ✓ A total of 11/3 cups of the meal.
- ✓ Take 1/2 cup of cooking oil.

Directions

1. Combine the paste of garlic, onion, paprika, salt, and pepper. Sprinkle the mixture over the tofu and apply gently.

2. In a large bowl, put the beer and add flour, stirring to mix.

3. Dip the tofu in the beer batter, fry on both sides until crispy in plenty of oil.

15. Casserole Polenta and Chili

Serving 4In 2 cups Calory: 405Fat: 7 grams Carbon: 59 g carbon: Protein: 16 g protein Fiber: 13 g fiber Sugar: 7 g.779 mg of sodium.

Ingredients

- ✓ 6 cups of vegetarian chili (about three cans if you buy from the store)
- ✓ 2 cups veggie mixture, any sort
- ✓ One cup of maize meal.
- ✓ 21/2 cups of water.
- ✓ Margarine 2 tablespoons vegan.
- ✓ 1 tablespoon chili powder

Directions

1. Combine vegetarian chili and vegetables and spread the casserole in the field.

2. Preheat to 375 ° f. Preheat oven.

3. Combine cornmeal and water in a saucepan over low heat. Simmer for 10 minutes, stirring sometimes. Stir in margarine vegan.

4. Disseminate the cornmeal mixture over chili and chili powder over the rim. Bake for 20–25 minutes uncovered

Chapter 4: Frozen Meals and Kids Friendly Recipes

4.1 Kids Friendly Foods

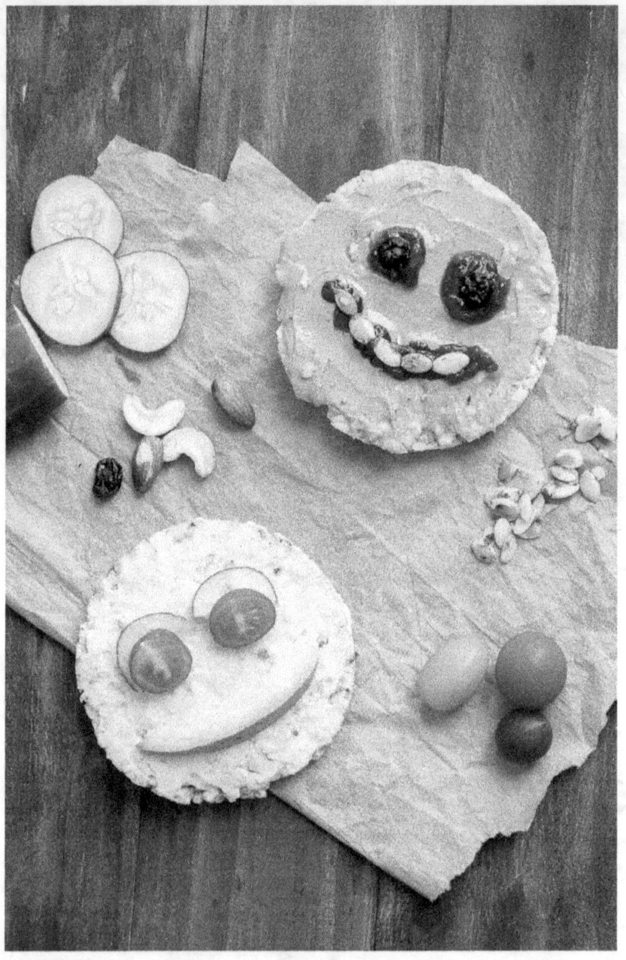

1. Sweetcorn & courgette fritters

Cook: 15 minutes

Serves 2 Nutrition: Kcal 465 kcal Fat 21 grams 5 g saturates Carbs 44 g carbs20 g sugars5 g optic Protein 23 g protein Salt 1.7 g salt

Ingredients

- ✓ 198 g can sweetcorn drained
- ✓ 2 spring onion, finely chopped
- ✓ 50 g zucchini, rubbed.
- ✓ 1 tsp smoked peppers
- ✓ 50 g of flour self-raising
- ✓ 5 eggs, 1 slaughtered, four poached.
- ✓ 40ml of milk
- ✓ 4 tbsp chili sauce
- ✓ Juice one lime
- ✓ 1 tbsp of vegetable oil.
- ✓ Mixed leaves

Directions

1. Stir in the large bowl sweetcorn, spring onions, zucchini, paprika, flour, beaten egg, milk, and seasoning.

2. Put on to boil a large saucepan of water. Mix the chili sauce and the lime juice in a bowl and set aside

3. In the four mounds of the fritter mix, heat the oil in a large, non-stick bowl and spoon separated (you can need to do this in two batches). Turnover and cook for 3 minutes, when brown on the underside.

4. In the meantime, poach the eggs 2-3 minutes in the water until the yolks are cooked and running. With a slotted spoon, remove. Serve the chips with a poached egg, mixed leaves, and a chili dressing drizzle.

2. Broccoli, Cheddar, and Brown Rice

Yield serving 4 (2 cakes serving size)

280 calories Fat 10.6 g fat5.2 g sat fat3 g mono fat1.1 g poly fat15 g protein-protein33 g carbohydrates g optic113 mg of cholesterol Iron 2 mg iron554 mg of sodium268 mg of calcium2 g sugars Added 0 g of sugar

Ingredients

- ✓ One tablespoon of unsalted butter
- ✓ 3/4 cup yellow chopped onion
- ✓ Four cloves of garlic, chopped.
- ✓ 3/4 cup of unsalted vegetable (like Swanson)
- ✓ 12 ounces of fresh broccoli, cut in 1/2-in.
- ✓ 1 (8.8-oz.) Pkg for pieces. Brown rice precooked (like uncle bens)
- ✓ 1/4 cup of whole wheat panko (Japanese breadcrumbs).
- ✓ One tablespoon of a mustard grain
- ✓ 1/2 teaspoon black pepper
- ✓ Kosher salt 3/8 teaspoon
- ✓ Cheese shredded sharp cheddar fat-reduced, divided (approximately 3/4 cup)
- ✓ 2 eggs, slightly beaten.
- ✓ 2 sliced green onions (optional)

Directions

1. Preheat 450 ° f oven. Preheat. Coat a baker with a spray for cooking.

2. Heat butter over the medium-high temperature in a large skillet. Add ointment and garlic. Sprinkle for 4 minutes. Incorporate stock and broccoli. Bring to a boil, cook for three minutes.

3. Heat rice according to the Directions of the box. In a large bowl, combine broccoli, rice, panko, mustard, pepper, salt, and 1/2 cup cheese. Remove the eggs. Divide into 8 (2 1/2-inch) pats and shape broccoli mixture. Arrange patties on prepared saucepan; spray coating patties on the cooking spray — Bake for 15 minutes at 450 ° f. Top the remaining 1/4 cup cheese and cook for another 4 minutes at 450 ° until the cheese melts. Add green onions if desired.

3. Crispy Summer Vegetable Baked Tacos

Prep time: 20 mins Cook time: 20 mins yield: 10-121xcategory: dinner.

Ingredients

- ✓ 1 teaspoon olive oil.
- ✓ 1 medium zucchini, diced.
- ✓ 1 medium squash, diced summer
- ✓ Diced one medium red pepper
- ✓ 1/2 little yellow, diced onion
- ✓ 1/2 teaspoon salt
- ✓ 1/4 teaspoon black pepper.
- ✓ 1 (15 ounces) of beans can be refreshed.
- ✓ 1 1/2 teaspoons of cumin ground
- ✓ 1 teaspoon powder of garlic.
- ✓ 1 tablespoon of peppers.
- ✓ 1/2 teaspoon (optional) smoked paprika.
- ✓ 10–12 tortillas of maize.
- ✓ Toppings: salsa, guacamole, Greek yogurt, cassava cream, hot sauce

Directions

1. 450 degrees f heat oven. Add olive oil, veggies, salt, and pepper in a large pot, Cook veggies 5-7 minutes until tender.

2. Add veggies and cooled beans and spices to a large mixing bowl. Mix until combined. Until combined.

3. Heat the maize tortillas just to soften (in the microwave or on the stovetop). Add approximately 1/4 cup of the bean mixture to half of the maize tortilla. Fold over the other half and pull it down to make sure all is closed.

4. Put the tacos on the large pot and bake, about 10 minutes, brown and crispy, and flip once.

5. Let your favorite toppings cool for a few minutes!

4. Muffin Box Pancakes

Preparation: 15 mins. Cook: 5 minutes

Serves 2 nutrition Kcal625 Fat21g Saturations6g Carbs78g Sucks17g Fiber16g protein23 g Salt 3.2 g

Ingredients

- ✓ 400g can kidney beans in spicy sauce
- ✓ 4 medium wraps of tortilla
- ✓ 400 g can be chopped green tomatoes.
- ✓ 230 g of green salad

Directions

1. Heat oven to fan / gas 6 200c/180c. In a pot, soak the beans and tomatoes for 15 minutes, then season.

2. In the meantime, grate a muffin tin with oil in four holes. Line each of them with a tortilla, make a cup, and fill with a foil ball.

3. Bake until slightly crisped for 5 minutes. Remove the foil, break the mixture among the cups of tortilla, and serve with a green salad.

5. Cheese Breadsticks

Serve 2 per 1/2 Calory: 194Fat: 4 g fat Carbon dioxide: 32 g Nutrition: 8 g protein Fiber: 2 g Sugar: 2.5 g Soy: 535 mg

Ingredients

- ✓ 1/2 tomatoes

- ✓ Four tablespoon vegan cream cheese
- ✓ 2 Tablespoon milk
- ✓ 1/2 teaspoon dried parsley flakes
- ✓ 12 pretzel sticks

Directions

1. Finely chop the tomato. To make the breadsticks dip, combine the cheese, the chopped tomato, the milk, and the parsley flakes.

2. Serve as it is or mixes the cheese for a smoother dip in the mixer.

6. The Supreme Pizza Cracker

Two serves Per three pizza wedges Calories: 178; Fats: 7.5 g Carbohydrate: 19 g Proteins: 8.5 g Fiber: 2 g Sugar: 2 g Sodium: 272 mg

Ingredients

- ✓ 2 tablespoons of tomato sauce
- ✓ 1 pita pocket
- ✓ 2 large mushrooms, sliced.
- ✓ Add two tablespoons of sliced olives.
- ✓ 1/3 cup of cheddar grated

Directions

1. Spread the tomato sauce over the pita bag. Attach the slices of the mushroom and the olives.

2. Sprinkle with the cheese over the top.

3. Broil for about 2-3 minutes, until the cheese has melted.

4. Cut up to 6 wedges.

7. Bars of Chewy Granola

Yields are about 16 bars.

For 1 bar Calories: 185 cm Fats: 12 g Carbohydrate: 16 g Protein: 5 g of Fiber: 2 g Sugar: 7 g Sodium: 10 mg

Ingredients

- ✓ 8 tablespoons of coconut oil
- ✓ 1/4 cup, plus two tablespoons of honey.
- ✓ 2 cups of rolled oats
- ✓ 2 tablespoons of toasted wheat germ
- ✓ 3/4 teaspoon ground cinnamon
- ✓ 1 tablespoon of sesame seeds.
- ✓ 2 eggs
- ✓ 1/2 cup raisins
- ✓ 1/2 cup of chopped peanuts.

Directions

1. Preheat the oven over a temperature of 300 ° f.

2. Heat the coconut oil with the honey in a small saucepan over low heat, stirring continuously.

3. In a large bowl, combine oats, wheat germ, ground cinnamon, and sesame seeds. Add the melted coconut oil and honey to the dry Ingredients and stir to blend. Add the Beaten eggs to the mixture, stirring to combine. Stir in the raisins and the peanuts.

4. Spread the mixture in a 9 "× 9" sized pan, press it down with a spatula and spread it evenly. Bake for about 15 minutes or until golden brown. Let it cool down and cut into bars.

8. Crispy Potato Pancakes

Serves four is for two pancakes Calories: 264; Fats: 2.5 g Carbohydrate: 54 g Protein: 8 g of Fiber: 4 g Sugar: 3 g of sugar Sodium 106 mg

Ingredients

- ✓ 1 egg
- ✓ 2 baking potatoes (such as Idaho russet), peeled.

✓ One medium-sized onion
✓ 1/8 teaspoon of sea salt
✓ One tablespoon flour (whole wheat)
✓ Coconut oil for frying

Directions

1. Eat the egg in a big bowl. Using the large-hole side of the rack, shred the potatoes into the longest shreds possible.

2. Grate the onion.

3. Remove the salt and sprinkle with the flour; combine with your hands.

4. Heat the oil until it shimmers but does not smoke (potato will shimmer at entry).

5. Shape eight pancakes out of the batter and fry them in 3 or 4 batches, squeezing out the excess water before slipping them into the pan.

6. Cook slowly, without moving for the first 5 minutes, then loosen with a spatula.

7. Switch after about 8 minutes, when the top appears to be 1/3 fried.

8. Finish cooking on the other side, about 4 minutes longer.

9. Drain the paper towels.

9. Fritos (Crisps of Cheese)

Serves four is Per 4 crisps Calories: 66 cm Fats: 5 g Carbohydrate: 0.5 g Protein: 5 g of Fiber: Sugar: 0 g of sugar Sodium: 382 mg of sodium

Ingredients

✓ 1 cup of finely chopped Parmigiano-Reggiano

Directions

1. Heat a non-stick skillet over medium heat.

2. Sprinkle one tablespoon of cheese in a medium saucepan.

3. Cook until the bottom is well browned, then move to the paper towels to drain.

4. They are soft and oozy and take a little practice to treat them properly, so have a little extra cheese ready if the first few are "less than perfect."

10. Salsa Fresca (The Pico De Gallo)

Serves 8 of for 1/4 cup Calories: 15 cm Fats: 0 g Carbohydrate: 3.5 g Protein: 1 g of Fiber: 1 g Sugar: 2 g of sugar Sodium: 141 mg of

Ingredients

- ✓ Four medium tomatoes, seeded and diced fine (about 11/2 cups)
- ✓ One small white onion, finely chopped.
- ✓ One jalapeno pepper, seeded and finely chopped.
- ✓ 1/2 teaspoon of salt.
- ✓ 2 teaspoons of lime juice
- ✓ 1/4 cup of minced cilantro

Directions

1. Purée one-third of the tomatoes in a blender or food processor.

2. Combine with the remaining tomatoes, cabbage, jalapeno, salt, lime juice, and cilantro. Better if used within two days.

3. Serve with chips, an omelet of cheese, or as a sauce with other Mexican foods.

11. The Spread of Vegan Chocolate Hazelnut

1 cup of yields

Calories: 148; Fats: 11 g Carbohydrate: 9 g Protein: 3 g Fiber: 3 g Sugar: 6g of sugar Sodium 1 mg

Ingredients

- ✓ 2 cups of hazelnuts, chopped.
- ✓ 1/2 cup of cocoa powder
- ✓ 1/2 cup of powdered sugar
- ✓ 1/2 teaspoon of vanilla
- ✓ 4 spoonsful of palm oil

Directions

1. Add hazelnuts, cocoa powder, sugar, and vanilla to the food processor and combine.

2. Add oil, just a little at a time, until the mixture is soft and smooth and the desired consistency is achieved. You can need to add more or less than four teaspoons.

12. Potato Pakoras (Fritter)

Serves 8 of for one fritter Calories: 86 cm Fats: 2 g Carbohydrate: 12 g Protein: 4 g ofFiber:3gSugar: 2 g of sugar Sodium: 158 mg of sodium

Ingredients

- ✓ 11/4 cups of chickpea flour
- ✓ 2 teaspoons of coconut oil
- ✓ 11/2 teaspoons of ground cumin
- ✓ 1/2 teaspoon of cayenne
- ✓ 1/4 teaspoon of turmeric
- ✓ 1/2 teaspoons of salt.
- ✓ 1/2 cup of cold water
- ✓ Oil for frying

Directions

1. 1 large or two medium-sized baking potatoes (about 8 ounces), peeled, then sliced into 1/8-inch pieces.

2. In a blender, pulse flour, olive oil, cumin, cayenne, turmeric, and salt 3 or 4 times until fluffy. Gradually add water with the blade spinning, then process for 2-3 minutes until smooth. Adjust the consistency by adding water until the mixture is slightly thicker than the texture of the cream. Cover and set aside for ten minutes.

3. Heat the oil to 350 ° f. Dip the potato slices in a batter one by one and put them in 6 or 7 pieces of fried oil. Fry on each side for almost 4–5 minutes, until golden brown and cooked through. Serve right away.

13. Ball of Vegan Cheese

Makes one big cheese ball or 12 pieces of cheese balls

Per 1 ball of cheese Calories: 130 cm Fats: 10 g Carbohydrate: 1 g Protein: 4 g Fiber: 1 g Sugar 1 g of sugar Sodium: 158 mg of sodium

Ingredients

- ✓ One block of vegan nacho cheese, room temperature
- ✓ one teaspoon of garlic powder.
- ✓ 1/2 tablespoon of hot sauce
- ✓ 1/4 teaspoon of salt.
- ✓ One jar of vegan cream cheese, room temperature
- ✓ One tablespoon of paprika
- ✓ 1/4 cup nuts, finely chopped

Directions

1. Grate the vegan cheese in a large bowl, or process in a food processor until finely chopped. Using a large fork, mash the vegan cheese with the cream cheese, garlic powder, hot sauce, and salt until well blended.

2. Chill until solid, at least 1 hour, then form a ball or log shape, press firmly. Sprinkle with paprika and roll over the nuts carefully. Serve with a cracker.

14. Tzatziki Vegan

11/2 cups of yields

For 1/2 cup: 75 calories Fats: 3 g Carbohydrate: 7 g Protein: 3 g Fiber: 1 g Sugar: 4 g of sugar Sodium: 10 mg of

Ingredients

- ✓ 11/2 cups of organic soy milk, simple
- ✓ One tablespoon of olive oil
- ✓ One tablespoon of lemon juice.
- ✓ Four cloves of garlic, minced.
- ✓ 2 cucumbers, grilled or finely chopped.
- ✓ One tablespoon of freshly chopped mint

Directions

1. Whisk together yogurt with olive oil and lemon juice until well blended.

2. Combine the remaining Ingredients.

3. Chill it for 1 hour before serving so that the flavors can be mixed. Serve in the rain.

15. Walnuts with Chocolate

1 cup of yields

For 1/4 cup Calories: 266; Fats: 19 g Carbohydrate: 21 g Protein: 5 g Fiber: 2 g Sugar: 18 g sugar Sodium: 9mmg

Ingredients

- ✓ 1/4 cup granulated sugar
- ✓ One tablespoon of honey
- ✓ 2 tablespoons of condensed milk
- ✓ 1 cup of walnut bits

Directions

1. In a medium-sized saucepan, whisk sugar, honey, and milk over low heat. Add the pieces of walnut, stirring to make sure they are entirely coated in a mixture of sugar. Heat on medium temperature and bring to a boil. Let it boil for a few minutes, occasionally stirring as the sugar darkens. When browned on the edges, remove from the heat.

2. Add the walnut mixture to the greased baking sheet and cool. Separate the walnuts and store them in an airtight container or plastic bag. (they 're going to last about a week)

4.2 Frozen Food Recipes

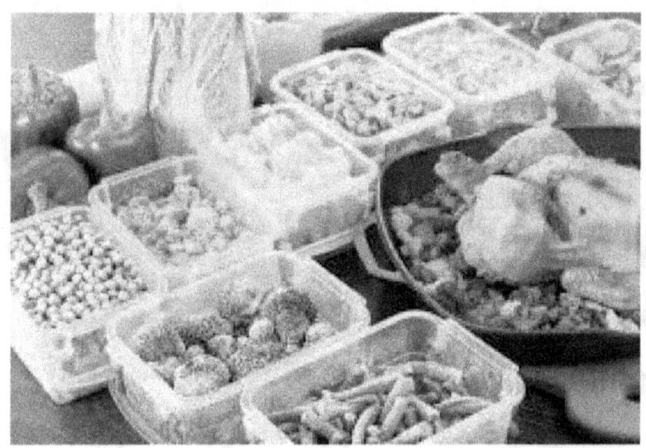

1. Healthy Kale and Lasagna Portobello

Overall: 1 hour 50 min, Prep: 25 minutes, Inactive: 15 minutes, Cook: 1 hour 10 minutes, Yield: eight portions

Ingredients

- ✓ One cup of drained jarred roasted red peppers coarsely chopped
- ✓ 1/2 teaspoon of oregano dried
- ✓ one 28-ounce tomatoes.
- ✓ kosher salt and black pepper freshly ground
- ✓ granular sugar for 1/4 teaspoon
- ✓ 1, and 1/2 cups of mozzarella cheese grated skim.

- ✓ 2 big white egg
- ✓ 15-ounce part-skim ricotta cheese container.
- ✓ one tablespoon of olive oil.
- ✓ The portobello mushrooms stalks discarded; 1/4-inch thick caps cut.
- ✓ 1 little bunch kale, discarded stems, coarsely chopped leaves.
- ✓ 1/4 teaspoon red pepper flakes crushed
- ✓ Two garlic cloves, thinly sliced
- ✓ non-stick cooking spray
- ✓ Nine sheets, such as barilla, no-boil lasagna noodles
- ✓ Two tablespoons of fresh parsley sliced poorly.

Directions

1. To 350 degrees f, preheat the oven. In a blender puree the peppers, oregano, onions, 1/4 teaspoon salt, 1/4 teaspoon pepper, and sugar until smooth and residual. Mix 1 cup of mozzarella cheese into a medium bowl with egg whites and ricotta cheese.

2. Heat the oil over medium-high heat in a large non-stick saucepan. Apply champagne and cook, stirring, until the liquid is released and tender, about ten minutes. Stir the pepper, garlic, and 1/4 teaspoon of salt in batches and continue cooking until the pepper is wilted and light green, another 5 minutes.

3. Nebulize a 9-by-13-inch bakery with a non-stroke spray. At the bottom of the dish, layer 3/4 cup of sauce. Two noodles, one half of the ricotta mixture, and one half of the mushroom mix. Repeat sauce layers, pasta, and other ricotta and mushrooms. Top with different noodles and sauce. Cover with aluminum foil and bake until tender noodles are bubbling around the edges of the pot, approximately 50 minutes.

4. Sprinkle it with the other 1/2 cup of grated mozzarella and bake for approximately five minutes until melting. Let stand for 15 minutes, sprinkle, and serve with parsley.

2. Salad Garden

Serving 1Per 1 dining Calory: 108Fat: 4 g fat: Carbon dioxide: 14 g Protein: 4 g proteinFiber:5gSugar: 8 g.382 mg of sodium.

Ingredients

- ✓ 4 iceberg leaves.
- ✓ 1/2 of tomatoes
- ✓ 2 celery stalks
- 1/2 cup of sliced champagne
- ✓ Quarter cup of carrots.
- ✓ 2 tablespoon low-calorie dressing salad

Directions

1. Wash the beans, onions, celery, and slice of lettuce. Wipe the champignons with a damp towel.
2. Half chop the baby carrots. Combine the salad Ingredients and dress in the salad.
3. Tip for vegetable cleaning
4. Please wash fresh food only before serving or feeding, even if you place it for the first time in the crisp portion of your refrigerator.

3. Fennel Rainbow Salad

Serving 2In 2 cups Calories: 190 calories Fat: 7 grams Carbon dioxide: 32 g Protein: 4 g protein Blueberry: 7 g Sugar: 15 g.260 mg sodium.

Ingredients

- One carrot.
- One red pepper bell
- 2 cups of red cod shredded
- Two tablespoons, plus two mayonnaise vegan teaspoons.
- Three teaspoons honey
- One bulb fennel

Directions

1. Wash the carrot and pumpkin gold. Grate the carrot (1/2 to 2/3 cup of grated carrot should be present) — thin strips of red pepper.
2. In a cup, combine the carrot, red pepper, and cabbage. Mix the mayonnaise with the honey. Toss the vegetables with the mixture of mayonnaise.
3. Rinse the fennel and dry it under running water. Cut off the fennel bulb top and bottom.
4. Cut the fennel into sections, remove the center of the heart and cut into small bits. Garnish the fennel with the salad.

4. Caesar Quick Salad

Serving 3By 1 cup. Calory: 176Fat: 10 grams Carbon dioxide: 13 g Protein: 7 g protein Cable: 3 g fiber Sugar: 4 g.340 mg sodium

Ingredients

- ✓ 3/4 roman head lettuce
- ✓ One big cup of croutons
- ✓ 1/4 cup of parmesan grated cheese
- ✓ Caesar salad dressing three teaspoons
- ✓ Black pepper

Directions

1. Wash the salad and dry the head. Cut the leaves in strips about 1 inch long.
2. Mix croutons, parmesan cheese, and lettuce together. Remove the Caesar salad dressing just before serving and sprinkle with black pepper.

5. Snow Peas Fruity

Serving 3Each one and a half cup. Calories: 80 calories Lip: 0 g Carbon dioxide: 13 g Nutrition: 2 g protein Fiber: 2 g Sugar: 5 g.10 mg of sodium

Ingredients

- ✓ 6 ounces of fresh snow fish
- ✓ 1/2 cup of cocktail juice canned fruit

Directions

1. Rinse in cold running water the snow peas. Drain and dry. Cut the ends.
2. In a shallow microwave-safe dish, put the snow peas and add the fruit cocktail juice.
3. 11/2–2 minutes microwave fire, or until the snow peas are fresh, luminous orange. Serve either hot or chilled. Serve.

6. Caramelized Carrots Baby

Serving 4By 1 cup Calories: 103 calories Fat: 5 grams Carbon dioxide: 12 g Protein: 1 g protein Cable: 3 g fiber Sugar: 8 g Soda: 302 mg

Ingredients

- ✓ 4 cups of sweet carrots
- ✓ One teaspoon citrus fruit juice
- ✓ Two tablespoons of margarine vegan
- ✓ One dough sugar brown
- ✓ 1/4 teaspoon salt or to taste

Directions

1. Soak carrots in the water for approximately 8–10 minutes until soft; do not overcook. Drain and rinse the lemon juice. Drain.
2. Heat carrots, margarine, brown sugar, and sea salt often stir until glaze is well coated and carrots about 5 minutes.

7. Whole Wheat Pasta with Tomato Pesto and Basil

Serving 2By 1 cup Calory: 479 Fat: 34 g Carbs: 34 g carbohydrates Protein: 13 g protein Fiber: 5 g Sugar: 3 g Sodium: 90 mg

Ingredients

- ✓ 1 cup of pasta rigatoni
- ✓ One ounce of fresh basil.
- ✓ 3 cloves of garlic
- ✓ 1 tomato
- ✓ 1/4 cup pine noodles
- ✓ 1/4 cup of parmesan grated cheese
- ✓ 1/8 taste of olive oil.

Directions

1. Cook pasta until tender but still firm in boiling salted water (al dente). Drain. Drain. Cut the basil leaves into 1 cup. Smash the garlic, peel, and chop. Wash the tomato and slice, conserve the juice.
2. In a food processor, process the pine nuts and garlic. Attach and prepare tomato and basil leaves one at a time. Apply olive oil slowly and continue to heat until the pesto is creamy. Remove the parmesan rubber cheese. Pour over the cooked pasta half the pesto sauce. Place the remaining pesto sauce in the refrigerator in a sealed jar for up to 7 days.

8. Spinach Noodles

Serving 2By 1 cup Calory: 243Fat: 16 g fat: Carbs: 19 g carbohydrate Food: 8 g protein

Fiber: 4 g fiber Sugar: 2 g.550 mg of sodium.

Ingredients

- ✓ 11/2 egg noodles cups
- ✓ Two garlic cloves
- ✓ Tomato 1
- ✓ One tablespoon olive oil

- ✓ 1 cup of frozen spinach thawed
- ✓ Two tablespoons of parmesan rated cheese
- ✓ 1/2 teaspoon of salt

Directions

1. Cook the noodles.
2. Thoroughly drain
3. Smash the garlic cloves, peel them and chop them. Slice tomato. Slice tomato.
4. In a pan, heat the oil over medium temperature. Add the tomato and garlic. Briefly cook, turn the heat to high and add the noodles.
5. Remove the spinach. Cook quite quickly, mix the spinach and the noodles and remove the oil. Remove the parmesan cheese — season as desired with salt.

9. Rice Coconut

Serving 4Tax: $1,56By 1 cup Calory: 343Fat: 6 g fat Carbon dioxide: 20 g Food: 8 g protein Fiber: 2 g Sugar: 3 g.310 mg of sodium.

Ingredients

- ✓ One cup of water
- ✓ One 14-ounce milk of coconut
- ✓ 11/2 tables of white rice
- ✓ 1/3 cup of flakes of cocoa
- ✓ One teaspoon-lime juice
- ✓ 1/2 teaspoon salt

Directions

1. Combine the water, coconut milk, and rice in a large pot and simmer. Cover and cook until rice is finished for 20 minutes.
2. Toast the cocoon flocks in a separate pot over low heat until slightly golden, approximately 3 minutes. Stir gently continuously to avoid fire.

3. Combine cocoa flakes with cooked rice and add salt and lime juice.

10. Italian Salad of Rice

Serving 6By 3⁄4 of a cup Calory: 212Fat: 10 grams Carbon dioxide: 25 g Protein: 4gproteinCable: 3 g fiber Sugar: 3 g.120 mg of sodium

Ingredients

- ✓ 1⁄3 cup of vinegar red wine
- ✓ One tablespoon of vinegar balsamic
- ✓ Two teaspoons of mustard Dijon
- ✓ 1⁄4 taste of olive oil.
- ✓ Four cloves of garlic, hairy
- ✓ One basil tablespoon
- ✓ Fresh parsley 1⁄3 cup chopped.
- ✓ 2 cups of rice
- ✓ 1 cup of green fish
- ✓ One carrot rubbed
- ✓ 1⁄2 cup of red pepper roasted, chopped
- ✓ sliced 1⁄2 cup of green olives.
- ✓ salt and pepper

Directions

1. Shake or whisk the red wine vinegar, balsamic vinegar, mustard Dijon, olive oil, garlic, basil, and parsley.
2. In a large bowl, mix rice with the remaining Ingredients. Toss well with dressing mix and coat.
3. Test, and season with a little salt and pepper.
4. Cool down for at least 30 minutes before serving so that the flavors can be set.

11. Parmesan Baked-Eggplant

Prep: 20 minutes Total: 1 hour 30 minutes Servings: eight

Ingredients

- ✓ Olive oil extra virgin, for brushing.
- ✓ 2 eggs
- ✓ Three-four cup dry breadcrumbs
- ✓ 3/4 cup parmesan finely rubbed and two teaspoons topped.
- ✓ One tablespoon of oregano dried.
- ✓ Dry basil with 1/2 teaspoon
- ✓ Kosher salt and pepper freshly ground.
- ✓ Two large eggplants (2 1/2 lbs.), peeled and cut into rounds of 1/2 inch.
- ✓ Six cups (48 ounces) of chunky tomato or homemade chunky tomato sauce, bought from the store.
- ✓ 1 1/2 cups of mozzarella shredded

Directions

1. Preheat the oven to 375 ° c. Brush 2 oil bakers; set aside. In a large dish, whisk eggs and two tablespoons of water together. Combine 3/4 cup of parmesan, oregano, and basil in another bowl; season with salt and pepper.

2. Dip eggplant pieces in the egg mixture, let the excess drop down, and then dredge in breadcrumb mixture, cover well. Bake on the bottom until golden brown, 20 to 25 minutes. Turn slices; bake for 20 to 25 minutes more until browned on the other side. Remove from oven; heat the oven to 400 ° c.

3. Spread 2 cups of sauce in a bakery 9-by-13-inch. Arrange half the eggplant with 2 cups of sauce and 1/2 cup of mozzarella. The rest of the eggplant, seasoning, and mozzarella, sprinkle with two other parmesan tablespoons. Bake for 15 to 20 minutes until the sauce is bubbling and cheese is melted. Enable 5 minutes to stand before serving.

12. Cannellini Beans Ratatouille

Serving 6By 1 cup. Calory:167Fat: 5 grams Carbon dioxide: 24 good: 8 g protein Fiber: 8 g Sugar: 8 g.405 mg of sodium.

Ingredients

- ✓ 2 teaspoons of olive oil.
- ✓ 1 onion, diced
- ✓ 2 turquoises, diced.
- ✓ 2 squash purple, diced
- ✓ 1 small aubergines, diced
- ✓ Diced 1 bell pepper
- ✓ 2 cups of cannellini, cooked
- ✓ One teaspoon flour
- ✓ Three tomatoes, seed, and cut into six sections
- ✓ Two teaspoons of dried herbs from Provence (including oregano, thyme, rosemary, marjoram, salivary including lavender combinations)
- ✓ One teaspoon salt
- ✓ Black pepper freshly ground.

Directions

1. In a heavy-bottomed Netherlands oven, heat the olive oil until hot but not smoky. Add onion; cook for about 5 minutes until translucent. Combine in a large bag of paper the zucchini, the yellow squash, the eggplant, and the bell pepper; dust with flour, fold bag closed, shake to coat. Add blurred vegetables, tomatoes, herbs, salt, and pepper to the pot.
2. Reduce heat to cook for 1 hour, cover, and cook carefully until all vegetables are tender. Serve hot or in the room.

13. Aubergine Rollatini

Serving 8Per 1 roller Calory: 339Fat: 13 grams Carbs: 34 g carbohydrates Protein: 22 grams Fiber: 6 g Sugar: 8 g856 mg of sodium.

Ingredients

- ✓ One large eggplant, cut into even 1/8-inch slices (as thick as a book cover) in the longitude.
- ✓ Meal to dredge

- ✓ Six beaten egg-washed, mixed with 1/2 cup water
- ✓ 2 cups of crumbs of bread
- ✓ Frying oil
- ✓ 1 pound of ricotta from
- ✓ 8 ounces of mozzarella ground cheese
- ✓ 1/2 cup of parmesan grated
- ✓ Salt and potato
- ✓ Fresh spinach, washed, and cooked 11/2 pounds.
- ✓ Tomato sauce 4 cups

Directions

1. Bread and fry the eggplant: dip one piece of eggplant into the flour, cover it on both sides; shake off excess flour, wash it in the egg, shake it out, and coat it into bread chips to keep it tightly. Place on a rack and repeat with remaining pieces. Heat oil to 350 ° f. Fry the breaded eggplant slices for almost 1 minute per side and drip off any excess fat before stuck between layers of towels.

2. Filling and rolling: 350 ° f heat oven. In a mixing bowl, combine the three slices of cheese and lightly season with salt and pepper. At the wide end of the fried aubergine, place one teaspoon cooked spinach and a generous teaspoon of cheese mix. Roll away from yourself, jellyroll, and put the seam on the bottom of the bakery. Repeat with remaining aubergines and fillings and close the finished roulades in a bakery.

3. Bake until the cheeses are hot, and the edges start to lightly brown. Serve with basil leaves in a bowl of tomato sauce — one piece per portion of aperitif, 2 per the main course.

14. Snow Peas and Mushrooms

Serves 4 • time preps: of 10 minutes

Ingredients

✓ 8 ounces of snow fish (approximately 3 cups)
✓ 8 ounces of mushrooms (about 8 ounces of cremini).
✓ one tablespoon cocoa oil.
✓ 1 cup of book choy chopped
✓ a quarter of a cup of sake (or dry sherry)
✓ 2 teaspoons raw or brown sugar
✓ 1 teaspoon gf tamari sauce.
✓ One tablespoon of sesame oil toasted
✓ 1/2 cup of bean spruce (optional)

Directions

1. Prepare the snow peas with the strings removed and halved diagonally. Clean the champagne and slice it into half if low or 1/2-inch slices if larger.

2. Heat a large skillet and add the cocoon oil over medium-high heat.

3. When the oil is soft, add the champagne and cook until its juices are released, frequently stirring, for approximately 3-4 minutes. Add snow peas and bokchoy and sauté for 1 minute.

4. Add sake, sugar, tamari sauce, sesame oil, and mix. Reduce the heat to medium-low and cook 2-3 minutes to blend the flavors. Serve immediately, if you like, topped by bean sprouts.

15. Black Chili Bean

Preparation: 10 mins. Cook: 30 minutes

Serves easy 4-6 Nutrition: Kcal339 Fat 10g Saturations1g Sugar 50g Suggestions 20g Fiber 8g protein 17g Sweet 1.45 g

Ingredients

✓ Take 2 pounds of olive oil.
✓ Cloves of garlic, finely chopped.
✓ Two big onions, chopped.
✓ A tbsp sweet chili powder or sweet pimento (Spanish paprika).

- ✓ 3 tbsp cumin ground
- ✓ 3 tbsp vinegar with wine
- ✓ Take 2 tbsp of brown sugar.
- ✓ take 2 x 400 g (2 x 14 oz) canes
- ✓ A double-four-hundred g (2 x 14 oz) can of black beans are rinsed and drained.
- ✓ Take some or one of the following to serve: feta-cheese crumbled, spring onion cut, sliced radishes, chunks of avocado, cream soured.

Directions

1. Heat oil in a big pot and then fry the garlic and onions for 5 minutes. Pimento and cumin are added, then cook for a couple of minutes, then add vinegar, sugar, tomatoes, and seasoning. Cook 10 minutes. Cook 10 minutes.

2. Pour in the beans and cook ten more minutes. Serve in small bowls with rice and accompaniments of your choice.

Chapter 5: Vegetarian Desserts, Snacks, and Sauces

5.1 Vegetarian Desserts

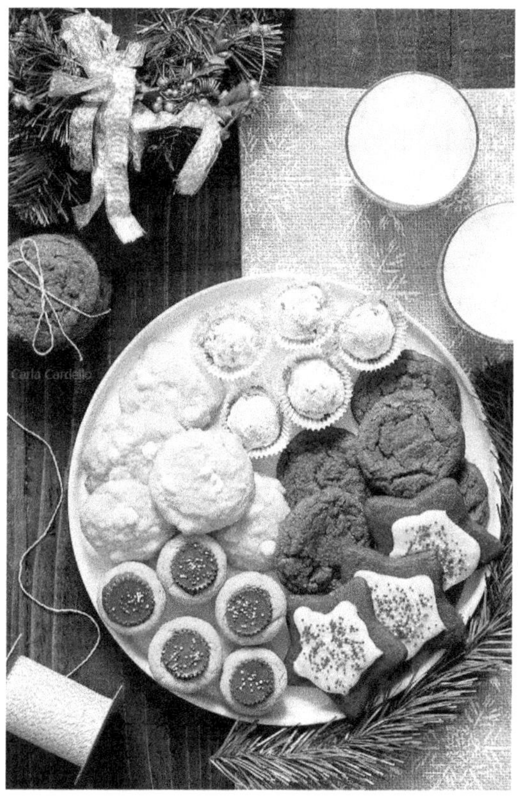

1. Speedy Mocha "Mousse" Pudding

Serves four is1/4 of the recipe Calories: 410 cm Fats: 31g Carbohydrate: 34 g Protein: 3 g Fiber: 2 g Sugar: 10 g of sugar Sodium: 270 mg of

Ingredients

- ✓ 2 cups of potent whipping cream
- ✓ 1/2 cup of instant coffee
- ✓ 1/2 cup of powdered sugar

- ✓ 1/2 cup of unsweetened cocoa powder
- ✓ One teaspoon of vanilla extract
- ✓ One instant vanilla pudding package
- ✓ 1/2 cup (or to taste) of prepared whipped cream
- ✓ Four cherries of maraschino

Directions

1. In a blender, combine the first six Ingredients. Mix at low speed (prepare in two batches if necessary). Dish in perfect glasses and let it sit for 5 minutes to allow the pudding to set. Add the whipped cream and a maraschino cherry to the top of each one.

2. Too much sugar can overwork your organs, leaving you tired and hungry, so make sure you only add it to your balanced diet in small amounts. The American heart association recommends nine teaspoons or 32 grams of sugar per day. The bottom line is to keep a treat, so enjoy the recipes in this chapter after you have consumed an adequate amount of protein and fiber.

2. Chocolate Fudge Mousse and Coffee Whipped Cream

Serves four of the recipe Calories: 310; Fats: 17 g Carbohydrate: 36 g

Protein: 6 g Fiber: 2 g Sugar: 5 g of sugar Sodium: 180mmg

Ingredients

- ✓ One package jello sugar-free and fat-free instant chocolate fudge pudding mix
- ✓ 2 cups of fresh skim milk
- ✓ 3/4 cup of heavy cream, chilled.
- ✓ 2–3 tablespoons of granulated sugar
- ✓ One tablespoon of prepared, robust coffee, chilled.

Directions

1. In a medium-sized mixing dish, combine the pudding mixture and the milk. I am using an electric mixer to beat

for around 11⁄2 minutes until the mixture is smooth. Divide the dough into four great cups as well. Set aside for 5-7 minutes.

2. Put the cream in a medium-sized mixing cup. Beat the cream until it's shaped. Sift the sugar over the cream and keep on beating it until soft peaks are formed. Stir in the coffee and combine until blended. Refrigerate until ready to be served.

3. To serve, top the pudding with the same amount of coffee whipped cream. Served to be chilled.

3. Banana Mouse

Serves six Per 3⁄4 cup of mousse Calories: 260 cm Fats: 22 g Carbohydrate: 16 protein: 2 g Fiber: 1 g Sugar: 9 g of sugar Sodium: 25 g

Ingredients

- ✓ Three big bananas, mashed
- ✓ 2 cups of whipping cream
- ✓ Three tablespoons of powdered sugar
- ✓ Two tablespoons of lemon juice
- ✓ 1⁄4 teaspoon (or to taste) of nutmeg ground
- ✓ One tablespoon of rum

Directions

1. In a blender, purée the bananas. Whip the cream at medium-high speed until high peaks are formed. Add the powdered sugar and whip briefly until soft peaks are formed (the mixture should be light and fluffy).

2. Fold the whipped cream to the mashed banana. Kindly whisk in the lemon juice, nutmeg, and rum. Put it in perfect glasses.

4. Easy Panna Cotta Italian

Serves five

It's a 4-oz. Serve Calories: 260 cm Fats: 22 g Carbohydrate: 12 g Protein: 3 g Fiber: 0 g

Sugar: 10 g Sodium: 40 mg of

Ingredients

- ✓ 1/4 cup of warm water
- ✓ One envelope of unflavored vegetarian gelatin, such as agar
- ✓ 11/2 cups of heavy cream
- ✓ 1/4 cup of granulated sugar
- ✓ Two teaspoons of vanilla extract
- ✓ 3/4 cup of milk

Directions

1. In a small bowl, add warm water. Add the gelatin over the water and let it melt for 5 minutes.
2. In a medium saucepan, bring the milk, sugar, and vanilla extract to a boil over medium heat. Reduce heat to low and simmer for 2-3 minutes, stirring regularly to ensure that all sugar is dissolved. Attach the milk and simmer for another 2-3 minutes.
3. Remove the saucepan from heat and pour in the softened gelatin (check to ensure that the mixture of cream and milk does not boil when you add the gelatin). Stir until the gelatin has completely dissolved.
4. In a pot, pour the mixture. Put the bowl inside another bowl of ice water. Cool for about 15 minutes, stirring regularly. Place the liquid in 4-ounce ramekins or custard cups and refrigerate overnight.
5. To serve, dip the bottom of each ramekin briefly in a bowl of hot water and use a knife to cut around the bottom of the panna cotta and loosen the edges. Dry the bottom of the ramekin and place the panna cotta on a plate. Enjoy as you are, or top with fresh seasonal fruit.

6. Considered to have originated in the piedmont district of northern Italy, panna cotta is Italian for "cooked cream." Traditionally, panna cotta is made from the vanilla bean. Still, the vanilla extract is a convenient substitute. Cut the grain in half lengthwise and scrape the seeds out if you want to add vanilla seed. Add both the bean and the seeds to the saucepan with the heavy whipping cream, stirring to ensure that the seeds are evenly distributed.

5. The Sundae Banana

Two serves1/2 Calories: 187; Fats: 1 g Carbohydrate: 45 g Protein: 3 g Fiber: 4 g Sugar: 29 g Sodium: 22mmg

Ingredients

- ✓ Two big bananas
- ✓ 1/4 teaspoon of ground cinnamon
- ✓ One teaspoon of cornstarch
- ✓ Two teaspoons of pineapple juice
- ✓ 1/4 cup of Greek almond yogurt
- ✓ 1/4 cup of crushed pineapple canned
- ✓ Two teaspoons of liquid honey

Directions

1. Peel the bananas and slice the hole lengthwise. Sprinkle with the ground cinnamon over the bananas. Mix the cornstarch in the juice of the pineapple and set aside.
2. In a small saucepan over medium-low heat, whisk yogurt, pineapple, and honey together.
3. Increase heat to medium and add the mixture of cornstarch and pineapple juice, whisking continuously until thickened.
4. Put the mixture over the bananas. If needed, sprinkle the extra cinnamon over the end.

6. A Shake of Creamy Tofu

Two serves for the 11/2 cups Calories: 255 cm Fats: 5 g Carbohydrate: 43 g Protein: 12 g of Fiber: 3 Sugar: 35 g Sodium: 65 g

Ingredients

- ✓ 101/2 ounces of light tofu
- ✓ 1 cup of frozen, unsweetened blueberries
- ✓ 1 cup of crushed pineapple canned with juice
- ✓ Two tablespoons of liquid honey
- ✓ 1/2 teaspoon of vanilla extract
- ✓ 1/3 cup of soy milk

Directions

1. Drain any excess water from the tofu and break it into pieces. If you use home-frozen blueberries instead of commercially purchased frozen berries, wash them before using them. Process the tofu and crushed pineapple with the pineapple juice from the can until it is smooth. Add the blueberries and process until it is smooth. Add the honey, vanilla extract, and soya milk and process again. Shake in the refrigerator until ready to Serve.

7. Oatmeal Supersized Cookies

Renders about 12 cookies

By one cookie Calories: 310 calories Fat: 18 grams Carbon dioxide: 37 g Protein: 3 g protein Fiber: 2 g Place of sugar: 23 g Soy: 160 mg

Ingredients

- ✓ 1/2 cup abbreviation
- ✓ 1/4 of a cup of sugar.
- ✓ 1 cup of brown sugar.
- ✓ One egg
- ✓ One tablespoon vanilla extract
- ✓ 1/2 teaspoon baking soda;

- ✓ 1/2 teaspoon oil!
- ✓ One cup of all-purpose meal.
- ✓ One teaspoon ground cinnamon
- ✓ 1 cup of fast-cooking oats
- ✓ Chips for 3/4 cup of semi-sweet chocolate
- ✓ 1/4 cup of walnuts chopped

Directions

2. Preheat the oven to 350 ° f. Preheat. Cream the shortening, butter and brown sugar together well. Beat in the extract of egg and vanilla.
3. Sift the salt and baking soda into the flour. Attach the cinnamon to the ground and blend well. Mix in the mixture of shortening and sugar. In the oats and chocolate chips, mix.
4. Shape into a ball about 2 inches in diameter 3 or 4 tablespoons of the pudding. Place on the bakery and separate well (6 balls to a bowl). Kindly press down with a fork. Place a few pieces of walnut in the center, if desired.
5. Bake for or until 13–15 minutes. Let cool in a jar that is airtight.

8. Muffins Banana Almond

Dairy right, gluten right

Prep: 5 minutes Cook: 15 minutes serving 6 minutes

Ingredients

- ✓ non-stick cooking spray
- ✓ 1 cup of almond butter
- ✓ 2 ripe bananas.
- ✓ 2 large eggs
- ✓ One tablespoon vanilla extract
- ✓ One teaspoon baking soda. One teaspoon
- ✓ 1/2 teaspoon with salt.
- ✓ 1/4 of a taste of milk-free chocolate chips.

Directions

1. Preheat the oven at 400 ° f temperature. Coat and reserve six muffin tin wells with cooking spray.

2. Combine almond butter, bananas, bacon, cinnamon, baking soda, salt, and chocolate chips in a strong blender. Pulse to blend for around 2 minutes.

3. Bake for twelve to fourteen minutes. The center is set when the tops come back when they are hit. Let the muffins cool in the pot for one week before being removed and stored in an airtight container.

Reheat:

If you want to eat them from frozen immediately, thaw in the defrost setting in the microwave for 1 minute.

Freeze:

You can also freeze those in a gallon-sized resealable freezer bag, individually wrapped in plastic, for up to 1 month — thaw for 1 hour at room temperature.

9. Buddies Skinny Muddy

Prep: 15 minutes Cook: 5 minutes serving 7 minutes

Ingredients

- ✓ 7 cups of wheat Chex cereal or other whole-wheat toasted cereal Chex
- ✓ 1 cup of dark chocolate chips
- ✓ 1/2 cup of natural creamy butter of peanut
- ✓ One tablespoon vanilla extract
- ✓ 1/3 cup of sugar powdered

Directions

1. In a big bowl, put the cereal. Set aside. Set aside.

2. Mix chocolate chips and peanut butter in a small microwave-safe bowl. In the microwave, heat up in 30 seconds, stirring until melted. Drop the coffee. Pour the mixture over the cereal and mix well. Transfer the cereal to a gallon-size resealable bag.

3.add the sugar powdered. Seal the bag and shake it. Divide the cereal into 1-cup portions in individual resealable bags — store for up to 1 week at room temperature.

10. No-Bake Butter Cookies

Dairy right, gluten right.

Prep: 15 minutes Cook: 5 minutes, plus 1-hour chill.

Ingredients

- ✓ 2 cups oats
- ✓ 1 cup of grossly chopped almonds
- ✓ Tablespoon of unsweetened cocoa powder.
- ✓ Take 1/2 cup of coconut oil.
- ✓ 1 cup of regular chunky butter of peanut
- ✓ 1/4 cup honey
- ✓ Two teaspoons of coffee.
- ✓ 1/2 teaspoon of salt.
- ✓ 1/2 cup dark chocolate chips

Directions

1. Remove oats, almonds, and cocoa powder together in a medium bowl. Set aside. Set aside.

2. In a small casserole, melt the coconut oil and the peanut butter over medium heat for three to four minutes. Remove the cup from the oven, add the honey and vanilla, salt and chocolate chips and stir until everything melts and melts. In the oat mixture, add this wet mixture and blend.

3. Using a small cookie scoop, make small, about two tablespoons of dough and place on a baking sheet. Placed the sheet about 1 hour in the refrigerator until the cookies are hardened.

4. Put three cookies into each of 5 resealable bags in quarter size. Suitable for up to 1 week. Freeze the remaining cookies for up to 1 month on potential snacks in a resealable gallon box.

11. Bites Dark Chocolate

Dairy-free, no-cook, dairy-free

Prep: 10 minutes plus 30 minutes to cool serve 5 minutes

Ingredients

- ✓ Two cups of fast cooking oats
- ✓ 1 cup of flaxseed field
- ✓ 1 cup of crunchy natural peanut butter
- ✓ Three scoops of protein chocolate powder (whey or vegan)
- ✓ Chips of 1/2 cup dark chocolate
- ✓ Six tablespoons of water or almond milk

Directions

1. Strip a bakery sheet or sheet of paper and set aside.
2. Combine the oats, flaxseed, peanut butter, protein powder, and chocolate chips in a medium bowl.
3. Add the almond milk and stir it until the batter is adhesive and rolls easily. Cut about 20 portions (approximately two tablespoons each) and roll into a disk. Place the balls on the pan prepared. Refrigerate until ready for 30 minutes.
4. Serve four bites in each of 5 resealable sandwich bags. Suitable for up to 1 week.

12. Vegan Fudge Foolproof

Renders 24 1-inch parts

Per 1-centimeter fudge Calories: 210 calories Fat: 12 g fat Carbs: 16 g carbohydrates Food: 2 g protein Fiber: 1 g fiber Place of sugar: 14 g.89 mg of sodium

Ingredients

- ✓ 1⁄3 cup of margarine vegan.
- ✓ 1⁄3 taste of cocoa
- ✓ 1/2 cup of soy milk
- ✓ 1⁄2 tablespoon of vanilla.
- ✓ Two cucumbers of peanut butter
- ✓ 3-31⁄2 cups of sugar powdered
- ✓ 3⁄4 cup nuts, neatly cut

Directions

- ✓ Grate a small bakery or square cake pan lightly.
- ✓ Melt vegan margarine with cocoa, soy, coffee, and peanut butter in a double boiler or over a low flame.
- ✓ Add powdered sugar gradually until the mixture is smooth, creamy, and thick. Remove in nuts.
- ✓ Move directly to the pan and chill until completely solid for at least 2 hours.

13. Frozen Dessert with Cappuccino

Serving 1 Calories: 160 calories Fat: 11 g Carbonates: 15 g Protein: 3 g Garlic: 0 g Sugar: 13 g 90 mg of sodium.

Ingredients

- ✓ 1 cup of cold coffee brewed
- ✓ Two tablespoon of cream cheese.
- ✓ One granulated sugar tablespoon
- ✓ Two teaspoon non-sweetened powder cocoa.

Directions

1. In a food processor, mix all the Ingredients until smooth.
    Freeze for 2 hours, sometimes stirring. Serve chilled.

14. Strong Strawberry

Serving 4 Calories: 190 calories. Lips: 4.5 carbon dioxide: 36
protein: 0 g protein Fiber: 2 g Place of sugar: 23 g Soy: 42 mg.

Ingredients

- ✓ Rinsed, dried, and hulled 1 cup of strawberries
- ✓ Greek yogurt 11/2 cups
- ✓ 1/2 cup of preserved strawberry
- ✓ Four whole strawberries, garnish
- ✓ Fresh mint leaves, to decorate

Directions

1. Divide the strawberries into four chilled martini glasses
    or ramekins in length.
2. In a medium-sized bowl, combine yogurt with
    strawberry preserves and mix until evenly mixed. Top
    with the mixture or using a piping bag with a rosette to
    cover each one. Garnish with a whole strawberry and a
    fresh sprig of mint.

15. Rice Coconut Pudding

Serving 4By 1 cunctatory: 448Fat: 20 tramcars: 60 g
carbohydrates Protein: 6 g protein Cable: 3 g fiber Sugar: 35 soy:
51 mg

Ingredients

- ✓ 11/2 cups of white rice cooked
- ✓ Vanilla soy milk 11/2 cups
- ✓ 11/2 cups of cocoa milk
- ✓ Three tablespoons of maple syrup.
- ✓ Two spoonsful of agave nectar
- ✓ Chopped 4 or 5 dates

- ✓ Cinnamon dash
- ✓ Two mangos, cut

Directions

1. Combine low heat rice, soy milk, and cocoa milk. Simmer very low for 10 minutes, or until thickening begins.
2. Mix in maple syrup, agave nectar, and heat for a further 2-3 minutes.
3. Enable to cool a little before serving, to thicken the pudding a bit. Just before serving, garnish with a splash of fresh cinnamon fruit.

5.2 Recipes of Snacks and Sauces

1. A Dip of White Bean

Makes 3 cups • prep time less than 5 minutes

Ingredients

- ✓ 11/2 cups of organic white kidney beans (or 1 [15-ounce] white kidney beans, drained and rinsed)
- ✓ 11/2 cups of organic garbanzo beans (or 1 [15-ounce] garbanzo beans, drained and rinsed)
- ✓ 1/4 cup of tahini sesame or sunflower butter
- ✓ 1/2 cup of freshly squeezed lime juice
- ✓ 1–2 tablespoons of olive oil
- ✓ One teaspoon of minced garlic (from 2 to 3 cloves of fresh garlic)
- ✓ 1/2 teaspoon of sea salt
- ✓ 11/2 teaspoons of hot or spicy paprika
- ✓ Two teaspoons of cumin
- ✓ 3–4 tablespoons of tamari sauce

Directions

1. Place all Ingredients in a food processor and pulse until entirely smooth. Place it in the refrigerator in a jar until ready to serve.

2. Breadsticks and Cheese

Two serves1/2 of the recipe Calories: 194; Fats: 4 carbohydrate: 32 protein: 8 g of Fiber: 2 sugar: 2.5 g sugar Sodium, 535 mg

Ingredients

- ✓ 1/2 of the tomato
- ✓ Four tablespoons of vegan cream cheese
- ✓ Two tablespoons of milk
- ✓ 1/2 teaspoon of dried parsley flakes
- ✓ 12 full-grain pretzel sticks

Directions

1. Finely chop the tomato. Mix the cheese, the sliced tomatoes, the milk, and the parsley flakes to make a dip for the breadsticks. Serve as it is or purées the cheese in a blender for a smoother dip.

3. The Supreme Pizza Cracker

Two serves Per three pizza wedges Calories: 178; Fats: 7.5 carbohydrate: 19 proteins: 8.5 g Fiber: 2 g Sugar: 2 g of sugar Sodium: 272 mg of

Ingredients

- ✓ Three tablespoons of tomato sauce
- ✓ One packet of pita
- ✓ Two large, sliced mushrooms
- ✓ Two tablespoons of sliced olives
- ✓ 1/3 cup of cheddar grated

Directions

1. Spread the tomato sauce over the pita bag. Attach the slices of the mushroom and the olives. Sprinkle with the cheese over the top. Broil for about 2-3 minutes, until the cheese has melted. Cut up to 6 wedges.

4. Bars of Chewy Granola

Yields are about 16 bars.

Calories: 185 comfits: 12 carbohydrate: 16 protein: 5 g of Fiber: 2 g Sugar: 7 g of sugar Sodium: 10 mg of

Ingredients

- ✓ Eight tablespoons of coconut oil
- ✓ 1/4 cup, plus two tablespoons of honey
- ✓ 2 cups of dried oats
- ✓ Two teaspoons of toasted wheat germ
- ✓ 3/4 teaspoon of ground cinnamon
- ✓ One tablespoon of sesame seed
- ✓ Three eggs
- ✓ 1/2 cup of raisins
- ✓ 1/2 cup of chopped peanuts

Directions

1. Preheat the oven to a temperature of 300 ° f.
2. Heat the coconut oil with the honey in a small saucepan over low heat, stirring continuously.
3. In a large bowl, combine oats, wheat germ, ground cinnamon, and sesame seeds. Add the melted coconut oil and honey to the dry Ingredients and stir to blend. Beat the eggs lightly and add them to the mixture, stirring to combine. Stir in the raisins and the peanuts.
4. Spread the mixture in a 9 "× 9" sized pan, press it down with a spatula and spread it evenly. Bake for about 15 minutes or until golden brown. Let it cool down and cut into bars.

5. Fritos (Crisps of Cheese)

Serves four Is Per 4 crisps Calories: 66 cm Fats: 5 g Carbohydrate: 0.5 g Protein: 5 g of Fiber: 0 g Sugar: 0 g of sugar Sodium: 382 mg of sodium

Ingredients

- ✓ 1 cup of Parmigiano-Reggiano finely chopped

Directions

1. Heat a non-stick skillet over medium heat. Sprinkle one tablespoon of cheese in a medium saucepan. Cook until the bottom is well browned, then move to the paper towels to drain. They are soft and oozy and take a little practice to treat them properly, so have a little extra cheese ready if the first few are "less than perfect."

6. Spinach and Artichoke Dips

12 serves

For 1/4 cup Calories: 90 cm Fats: 7 g Carbohydrate: 4 g Protein: 6 g of Fiber: 2 g Sugar: 2 g of sugar118 mg sodium

Ingredients

- ✓ Two 15-ounce cans quartered artichoke cores, drained and rinsed.
- ✓ One red pepper, finely chopped
- ✓ One green pepper, finely chopped
- ✓ One bag of 10 ounces of frozen spinach
- ✓ Three cloves of garlic, minced
- ✓ 1 cup of plain Greek yogurt
- ✓ 8 ounces of cream cheese
- ✓ Black chili pepper
- ✓ 1/4 cup of parmesan cheese

Directions

1. Preheat the oven on a temperature of 325 ° f. Mix all Ingredients except parmesan cheese. Spread in a 9 "× 9"

baking dish or an 11/2-quarter casserole dish, sprinkle parmesan over the top and bake for 30 minutes until golden brown. Serve with whole-grain crackers and raw vegetables.

7. White Bean Spicy – Citrus Ip

Serving 12Per one and a half cup. Calories: 70 calorie Fat: 0.5 g fat Carbons: 12 g carbohydrates Protein: 4 g protein Fiber: 4 g fiber: Sugar: 3 g. Soy: 257 mg

Ingredients

- ✓ Two 15-ounce buckets of dry, drained, and rinsed beans.
- ✓ 1/4 cup of simple Greek yogurt
- ✓ One orange zest rubbed
- ✓ One tablespoon mashed chipotle.
- ✓ One teaspoon-lime juice
- ✓ 1/4 teaspoon salt.
- ✓ 1/2 cup of a white onion diced
- ✓ One tablespoon of coriander chopped.

Directions

1. In the food processor, puree the beans, Greek yogurt, orange zest, chipotle purée, lime juice, and salt until smooth. Attach the onions and cilantro; blend with the rubber spatula.

8. Parsley and Dip Onion

Serving 61/4 of a cup. Calory: 54Fat: 3 grams Carbon dioxide: 4 g Protein: 5 g protein Fiber: 1 g Sugar: 2 g.104 mg of sodium.

Ingredients

- ✓ One onion, sliced
- ✓ Three cloves of garlic, medium
- ✓ One tablespoon olive oil
- ✓ One corporate tofu block, well pressed
- ✓ 1/2 teaspoon paste of onion.

✓ Three cucumbers with citrus juice
✓ 1/4 cup of fresh chopped parsley
✓ Two tablespoons of fresh chives chopped.
✓ 1/4 tablespoon salt.

Directions

1. Sprinkle onions and garlic in olive oil for 3–4 minutes until onions are tender. Remove from heat and slightly cool.
2. Treat onion and garlic in food processors with tofu, onion powder, and lemon juice until the onion is hacked and the tofu is almost smooth.
3. Mash the rest of the Ingredients by hand.

9. Pecans Spiced

Renders 3 cups Per one and a half cup. Calory: 209Fat: 21 grams Carbon dioxide: 4 g Protein: 3 g protein Fiber: 3 g Sugar: 1.5 g.128 mg of sodium

Ingredients

✓ Unsalted butter 1 ounce (2 tablespoons)
✓ 1-pound whole, pecans shelled
✓ Dark soy sauce two tablespoons
✓ One tablespoon hoisin sauce
✓ Hot pepper sauce a few drops

Directions

1. Preheat the oven at 325 ° f. Melt butter in a big pot. Add nuts, fry, throw, occasionally, until nuts are well coated. Attach a sauce of soy, hoisin, and hot pepper sauce; cook another 1 minute. Remove thoroughly to cover.
2. Spread the nuts over a baking sheet in a single layer. Bake to remove the liquid and brown the nuts. Switch off the oven. The calm before serving. Before serving.

10. Pecans Glazed

Renders 1 cup1/4 of a cup Calory: 257Fat: 22 grams Carbon dioxide: 15 g Protein: 3 g protein Fiber: 3 g Sugar: 12 g.2 mg of sodium.

Ingredients

- ✓ Unsalted butter two tablespoons
- ✓ Cup 1/8 brown sugar
- ✓ One tablespoon honey
- ✓ One teaspoon cinnamon ground
- ✓ 1 cup of sin.

Directions

1. Heat the butter in a small saucepan. Add brown sugar, honey, and ground cinnamon. Stir in the mixture and substitute the pecan.
2. Turn the heat on medium temperature and boil until the brown sugar is dissolved.
3. Place the pecan mixture on a grated pan and cool. Separate and store in a container or plastic bag that is airtight. (they're going to last approximately one week.)

11. Spiced Noodles

Renders 4 cups Per one and a half cup. Calory: 266Fat: 24 grams Hydrates of carbohydrates: 10 g Protein: 5 g protein Fiber: 2 g fiber Sugar: 7 g. Soy: 1 mg.

Ingredients

- ✓ Two half cups of walnut
- ✓ Four unsalted butter tablespoons
- ✓ Four cubs of raw sugar
- ✓ Two teaspoons of powder with five spices

Directions

1. Preheat oven to 350 degrees Celsius.

2. Place the walnuts on an ungrated bakery plate. Toast for 8–10 minutes and often check at the end of the baking time to ensure that they do not burn.
3. While the nuts are toasting (approximately 2 to 3 minutes before completion), melt the butter in the pot at low heat. Stir in the sugar to dissolve. Stir in the powder of five spices.
4. Stir in the toasted nuts and cover. Briefly cook until the liquid is completely absorbed. Place the walnuts on the baker's sheet and separate. Let cool.

12. Walnuts Caramel

Renders 1 cup1/4 of a cup. Calory: 266Fat: 19 g carbohydrates Protein: 5 g protein Fiber: 2 g fiber Sugar: 18 g sodium 9 mg

Ingredients

- ✓ 1/4 cup of sugar granulated
- ✓ One tablespoon honey
- ✓ Two tablespoons of condensed milk without sweetening
- ✓ 1 cup pieces of walnut

Directions

1. Remove sugar, honey, and milk over low heat in a medium-sized pot. Add the walnut pieces and swirl to ensure that they are fully coated in the sugar mixture. Increase heat to medium and boil. Stirring occasionally, let boil for several minutes, as the sugar darkens. Remove from the heat if it has browned on the edges.
2. Put the walnut blend in a greased bakery plate and cool. Break the walnuts and store in a jar or plastic bag that is airtight. (they're going to last approximately one week.)

13. Spicy Dip Black Bean

For the minutes over 3 cups, time preps 5 minutes.

Ingredients

- ✓ Two cups of organically cooked black beans (or two cans of black beans, drained and rinsed)
- ✓ Take cloves of garlic, chopped
- ✓ 1/2 cup fresh cilantro chopped
- ✓ Freshly squeezed lime juice for tablespoons.
- ✓ One teaspoon ground cumin
- ✓ 1-2 teaspoons red pepper flakes red pepper
- ✓ 1/4 teaspoon ground cinnamon;
- ✓ 1/4 teaspoon sea salt
- ✓ Pepper to taste

Directions

1. In a meal, combine all the Ingredients
2. Blend until creamy and smooth.
3. Add salt and pepper to it.
4. Serve with vegetables or Chips.

14. Alfredo Sauce

Non-Dairy

Serves 4 time prep: on 5 minutes.

Ingredients

- ✓ 2 cups of raw macadamia nuts
- ✓ Take 1 cup of cashew milk (page 198) or store-bought dairy (e.g., almond)
- ✓ 2 tablespoon green onions/scallions chopped.
- ✓ One tablespoon of garlic chopped.
- ✓ 1/2 tablespoon of salt.
- ✓ 1/2 teaspoon nutmeg.
- ✓ Two tablespoon mock parmesan cheese
- ✓ Two tablespoons of nutritional yeast.
- ✓ To taste salt and fresh cracked pepper

Directions

1. Pulse a food processor with macadamia nuts

(or blender) until it is like an excellent meal for consistency. Add the remaining Ingredients (except salt and pepper) to the food processor and whirl until the mixture is creamy and smooth, and all the Ingredients are fully integrated.

2. Take out the food processor and season to taste with salt and pepper. Serve your favorite noodles with the sauce. Add additional cheese to the dish, if desired. Place what remains in a jar that is airtight for 2-3 days in the fridge.

15. Tahini Sesame and Lime Dressing

Makes 1 cup prep time: less than 10 minutes

Ingredients

- ✓ 2 teaspoon of Dijon mustard
- ✓ 2 tablespoons of tahini sesame
- ✓ 2 tablespoons coconut cream (or canned coconut milk, full fat)
- ✓ Three tablespoons of grapeseed oil
- ✓ Add 1/4 cup of freshly squeezed lime juice.
- ✓ two teaspoons of kelp granules (optional)
- ✓ 3/4 teaspoon of sea salt
- ✓ fresh cracked pepper to taste.

Directions

1. Place all Ingredients in a blender or food processor and whirl to fully incorporate — season with salt and fresh cracked pepper to compare. Put the dressing in the refrigerator in an airtight jar.

Conclusion

You should not only understand what the vegetarian diet is after reading this book, but it can do it for you. This diet is nothing in the market like fad diets: it is a balanced lifestyle decision that will transform your life entirely. You will significantly reduce the chances of certain diseases, including type 2 diabetes, heart disease, and even cancer, by removing meat from the diet.

The vegetarian diet has a variety of advantages, so you don't have to pick only one as your reason to switch on it. Food gives more than pure calories to the body. This will improve or exacerbate your health, depending on what comprises your diet. Eating healthy is indeed one of the most important keys to a long and healthy life. This is, therefore, worth understanding that food can never be used as a supplement to traditional medicine. Now you are prepared to embark on a new adventure-vegetarian lifestyle by utilizing the knowledge you gained in reading this book, as well as the recipes you have given!